Quit Drinking

Easy Step By Step Guide to Stop Drinking Alcohol and Delete it From Your Life

Allen Grace

held against the publisher for any reparation, damages, or monetary loss due to the information herein, either directly or indirectly.

Respective authors own all copyrights not held by the publisher.

The information herein is offered for informational purposes solely, and is universal as so. The presentation of the information is without contract or any type of guarantee assurance.

The trademarks that are used are without any consent, and the publication of the trademark is without permission or backing by the trademark owner. All trademarks and brands within this book are for clarifying purposes only and are the owned by the owners themselves, not affiliated with this document

II

Table of Contents

Introduction

How much do you drink? As a rule, when answering this question, people begin to describe how they drink: "well, on holidays, however, they have now made a lot of holidays", "only beer, never vodka - only alcoholics drink vodka", "only in company, because you can sleep alone nicely afterward!"

It is strange that our perception sees exactly this side of the problem. People around and even some experts also start a conversation with these signs. Quite a detailed description of binges. Regular fractional use often causes controversy. Opinions are expressed about the benefits or harms of such use. There are pseudo-recommendations on how to determine whether a person is an alcoholic or not.

When contacting a doctor, patients, and their surrounding people thoroughly tell what kind of drinks, when, and under what circumstances a person took alcohol. It can be seen that they prepared for this story in advance, considering it to be important.

This is the main mistake! It is important to understand how a person drinks does not have much practical significance. The nature of the binges can be used to judge the condition of the liver, stomach, heart, and other internal organs. This is undoubtedly important information. Let us look a little deeper into this, shall we?

It should be noted that the main problem is not in the internal organs, but in the soul. The trouble of a dependent person is that he cannot help but drink. It is useless to discuss where the rake struck if we cannot understand why the person continues to attack drinks.

How often do you see the bewilderment of resuscitation doctors who treated a person two months ago after a severe complication of a binge, struggled for his life for a long time, was saved, and a month later, he again comes to them with the same diagnosis. This disease develops in a sober state until the person is drunk. After the first sip, everything will be "clear." Although the main focus, for some reason, is given to drinking bouts.

It is extremely important to immediately explain: binge is only a manifestation of a disease, one of many manifestations. Yes, of course, this is the most dramatic sign, but alcoholism is a condition that leads to binges.

While a person behaves strangely, suffers a hangover and torments others, friends, relatives gather, call a doctor. But as soon as it was all over - the topic closes, the patient does not want to talk about it, and everyone does not want to provoke a reminder. The most convenient way to "solve" a problem is to pretend that it does not exist...

Most patients, having gotten out of excess, make an oath promise: "That's it! This time is the last; this will not happen again. "

People often believe.

Firstly, I really want to believe. After all, this promise 100% coincides with the desire of others. Secondly, the promise sounds extremely convincing; at such moments, the patients really speak emotionally and reasonably; it is clear that the person is not joking and is not going to deceive.

What horror the family will experience when, after some time, everything will be repeated again. Alcoholics are beginning to be blamed for the fact that they are inveterate deceivers, they all lie. This is partly true, with the only difference being that an alcoholic, like any other dependent person, is a specialist in deceiving himself. He did not lie when he promised that he would not drink more; he really believed in what he was saying. He had a very clear and clearly formed opinion.

It remains only to answer the question: Why is this happening?

Yes, talking with the patient about the disease itself is a good idea. However, and quite understandably, it sometimes seems that his intellect is not all right. But this does not mean that this person cannot be at the same time the head of a large organization or a prominent scientist. Primitively, he only talks about drinking, but if he is asked about something else, you begin to make sure that he is not so stupid.

Regarding life experience, it is also not so simple. Still, these people are middle-aged and older, and have seen a lot and understand a lot.

On willpower in general, a separate conversation. As a rule, alcoholics are very strong-willed people. Well, just imagine, what willpower must be possessed in order to risk your health and life so, starting to drink, remembering how it ended the last time? One patient said so: "You see, doctor. I have strength and will. But there is no willpower!"

So what happens in the soul of an alcoholic before the first sip of alcohol, from which another binge begins?

This disease is very tricky. It does not damage the intellect, not life experience, and not willpower. It hurts the mind itself! That is what all of these tools in this book will work for.

In just two or three weeks, it begins to seem that the last binge was not a nightmare, but an adventure. Well, maybe too extravagant, but still an adventure. "... Of course, you can't drink like you did last time! But, in principle, if neatly, correctly, so as not to harm anyone, then why not?"

People laugh at themselves, wondering how quickly all the bad things were forgotten. It seems to them that they have some kind of short memory. You can, of course, consider this as well, but an alcoholic is a person has not forgotten but changed his mind! Within a month - another begins to seem that drinking is not only possible but also necessary! The man is sure that it is today, and right now that you need to drink a little, that this time, there will be no binge. He believes that there was no need to drink yesterday, and most likely, he will not drink tomorrow. He has an opinion that he fully controls the process and "can afford it."

The most commonly used phrase in this state is: "Well, sometimes I can't drink it! I'm my own boss, I want - I drink, I want - I don't drink!"

Forgetting is a natural process; we all sooner or later forget a lot, but changing the mind to the opposite is no longer in itself a personal decision.

Imagine a ball rolling on a table. It has stopped. This is understandable; it had to stop sometime. But, suddenly, the ball went in the opposite direction. It itself could not change the direction of movement, which means there is some kind of force; there is someone or something that made it roll there. This force in humans is called addiction, which makes sense to talk about.

It turns out that addiction is what happens in a sober state before drinking. To the first glass, bottle, mug - to the first sip of alcohol.

Dependence is a mental process, and therefore there is no, and there will never be such analyzes, according to the results of which the doctor will be able to show this process. Imagine a study such as an analysis of a person's thoughts, followed by printing on paper! Of course, there are no such devices and are unlikely to ever appear. Thoughts are something so scary that I personally would not want to see such equipment in action. There is an x-ray of the head, but there is no picture of the soul in which you could show a dark spot and say, "you see, this is an addiction."

The greatest insidiousness of this condition is that it is not felt.

In fact, it can be a parasitic disease. After all, an alcoholic is a person who feeds his illness himself. It is he who spends his health, time, self-respect to feed his addiction. Any parasite begins with the fact that it anesthetizes the site of the bite. A person feels cravings, intoxication, and a hangover, but dependence is not felt. And therefore, out of hard-drinking, an alcoholic cannot understand why he is considered sick? Well, in fact, because nothing hurts, doesn't hurt, and the medical board recently passed - they said that everything was within the normal range.

Yes, the situation is unusual: no one can prove anything, and the patient himself cannot feel anything. How to be back to sanity?! The only way out is to give a person the opportunity to make a choice, make a decision: all this happens against my will, which means illness. Same as cough or runny nose. Neither intellect nor willpower can stop either the first or the second.

Or: it happens according to my will. Then we are talking about pranks, licentiousness, a strange way to have fun, etc. Probably, such a person lives incorrectly. But does anyone know what is right? This is a question from the field of morality, ethics. A doctor definitely should not teach anyone how to live. It is important to understand that the choice is only between two either - or. There is no third option. Only one who made the first choice can change something in his life.

You cannot help a person who is confident that he does not need help.

Chapter **1**:

Illness or Weakness?

If a person nevertheless admits himself sick, and we see that this can only be admitted by yourself, then such a person can abandon the feeling of shame for what happened. Alcoholism is a disease of altered morality. After a binge, a person is immensely ashamed of what happened. People are surprised; why wasn't it a shame while drinking? Under the influence of craving, it was also embarrassing, but "craving" (the medical term - compulsive drive) is regarded by a sick mind as one of the natural needs. The ancient mechanism comes into force: "ashamed, but what to do?" After getting intoxicated, the shame goes away completely. Man is already becoming another creature. But after a binge, the feeling of shame is double.

When ashamed of a problem, patients lose the opportunity not only to solve it but even to ever begin to solve it. It is impossible to cope with what you are ashamed of. An alcoholic is like a person sweeping cockroaches under a sofa, just to not see them. He will be forced to cover this topic of conversation all his life either with silly laughter (often you have to see adults begin to giggle like schoolchildren when this topic is mentioned), or theorizing (resonant reasoning about the philosophy, biochemistry and historical roots of the process), or simply gross denial. One way or another, but after two or three phrases, you'll have to hear something like: "Well, okay, enough about that!"

People involved in the fate of the patient, also do not really like to talk about this topic. They believe that once again, it is not worth provoking. The man already looks repentant. Yes, and they themselves do not like it, it is better to forget and live on.

However, forgetting will not work, not only because it is impossible to forget, but also because soon it will happen again. And again, we will treat the consequences without affecting what causes them.

If an alcoholic pleads ill, then the feeling of shame becomes surmountable. No need to be ashamed of disease. After all, no one is ashamed of bronchial asthma or hypertension. Yes, you can't talk to everyone about this topic. Many will react incorrectly, but it is not necessary for everyone.

- There are relatives, close people who already know everything, and if they don't know something, "tell about yourself" is a normal phrase with close relations.

- There are people who have dealt with this problem. They will react correctly; they will neither laugh nor be rude. A conversation with such a person is extremely useful. Many of them want to share their experiences and will be grateful to those who want to listen to them.

- Finally, there are doctors, to understand the patient and show compassion for him is their professional duty. It is foolish to be ashamed of a doctor. In any case, if you do not step over the feeling of shame, you will not succeed at all. You do not get off the ground what you stand with your back to.

By admitting that he is ill, a person can give up the guilt. True, to refuse does not mean to lose. These feelings will not go away immediately and not forever. The important thing is that the patient ceases to take them into account in his logic. He understands that these are painful feelings. This is how his illness hides from him. Yes, alcoholism is a psychiatric illness, madness. But the madman is not guilty.

An alcoholic really feels eternally guilty. Sometimes, he even thinks that it's good that it will help him stop drinking. Others, as a rule, cultivate this feeling with good intentions, believing that this will bring the patient closer to sobriety, to treatment. It is customary to report the patient, scold, point out to him his shortcomings, in a word, to educate him as a small child. The effect is actually quite the opposite!

Firstly while a person considers himself guilty and not sick (and these are conflicting concepts), he will involuntarily seek excuses. An alcoholic turns into an unfortunate person who protects the one who kills him – alcohol. He is forced to constantly explain to himself and everyone why he drank? Alcoholic alibis begin to be built, one more ridiculous than the other (such a life, such a job, such a wife, etc.). People around start to argue on this subject: "it's not so bad, you couldn't even drink as I do." These disputes are endless and useless. There are no excuses because there are no accusations: Either you consider yourself sick - yes, this is insanity, but it is a disease, then the disease is to blame. No one is justified in the fact that he has a toothache, or there was an attack of radiculitis. Or you can retain your belief that it's not a disease, then it means that you live like that. Yes, we don't like it, but what you can do is your choice...

No one needs to theorize why a thief came and stole everything. Yes, because he is a thief! The question is, why it penetrated so easily? So there was no protection.

Secondly, as long as a person considers himself guilty, he will consider that they are offered not help, but punishment. If you are guilty, then they are punished! For the time being, an alcoholic refuses all manipulations and influences. He cannot afford help because he considers himself "not guilty enough." All talk on this topic is annoying. The perception of the topic is changing: advice is perceived as reproaches, jokes, as a mockery, the very word "alcoholic," invariably, as an insult.

"Why bother me?" is a very common question at this stage. One would like to answer: "why does a person go to the dentist?" It may even hurt there, but they don't drag him there by force, patients themselves turn. Such logic lasts until the guilt becomes so painful that it will be easier to get punishment. The punishment itself becomes desirable; it relieves for a time of guilt. After all, they're not punished twice. I drank again - and the topic was closed at a hospital once more.

The "poor fellow" did the procedure, and then the nightmare begins: we are so arranged that we cannot get what we did not expect. Once I went for punishment at the hospital - I received the punishment. This patient will be tormented all this time, suffer, torment himself and others, he should be bad - because he was punished! Sometimes, by the end of the year, the family begins to whisper: "He will definitely drink as soon as the treatment ends. Another drink! He pulled the emotional spring for a whole year, and now he let go ..." These events are part of alcohol mythology; everyone heard about a friend or relative who had everything turned out just like that. Such a result cannot be considered positive; it is only a change in the frequency of disruptions, and even then not always. This does not mean that you do not need to seek help. It is important to understand that the result is 90% dependent not on the method, but on what the patient himself was oriented to. If he is to blame, it means punishment; if he is sick, it is help, deliverance, after which he will become better.

Thirdly, as long as the alcoholic considers himself not sick, but guilty, he will be forced to make amends until he drinks. This is the curse of alcoholics - people who live on hard drinking. They not only drink heavily but also work, read, love impulsively, as if it was another binge for them. Jumping out of an alcoholic nightmare, experiencing an immense sense of guilt, such a person begins to involuntarily search for a feat. He needs exorbitant fatigue because only extreme fatigue will help get rid of guilt. How often you hear from patients: "Well, what an alcoholic I am, I work!"

Of course, you work, how you work! After all, you need to feed not only yourself but also your alcoholism. Unfortunately, thoughts will be. After all, we are talking about a disease, and it will develop. Increasing momentum, sooner or later, such a patient still reaches a certain limit of fatigue, and then another breakdown begins. This is a vicious circle, or rather a spiral leading down. In this arena, people move like circus horses for years and decades. Alcoholism is a very cunning host. He is not interested in the quick death of his slaves. Therefore, alcoholics live relatively long. If nothing bad happens - trauma, poisoning, and other causes of early mortality - an alcoholic can live up to 60 and 70 years. The truth is that all this time, he does not live, but feeds the disease. He studies, marries, has children, but all his life he is in two states - either unconsciously preparing for a binge, or is in it. There is only one way to jump from this carousel of madness - to admit that you are sick. In this case, sobriety is not a way to make amends, but a way to begin to live as intended. Each person was born for happiness, but an alcoholic cannot afford it.

While an alcoholic drinks, he dooms himself to an existence in which he is either unhappy or drunk. In sobriety, the alcoholic must be happy. Otherwise, he will get drunk - this is not a wish, but a medical recommendation, the possibility of saving a life!

By admitting that he is sick, a person can abandon feelings of shame and guilt. He can exchange them for dignity.

Sobriety is a virtue for those who understand. There is such a variation in this feeling. Do not be offended by a friend who, in response to a confession: "I haven't been drinking for six months," answers: "so what?" If you happen to talk to a person who has not been drinking for five years, he will answer something like: "I remember the first six months ... Well done, come on, keep t up!

This is real pride, not pompous, but special. Forgive those who do not understand this. Many of them are not alcoholics, they do not understand, and they do not need to understand this. And many of those who do not understand are sick people who still have not admitted this to themselves. We will pity them, God willing, and they will someday receive this pride.

The most important conclusion from recognizing yourself as a patient is a desire to stop drinking alcohol forever. That is, for life, any alcoholic beverage, in any quantity for any reason. In this case, we are talking about absolute sobriety.

In narcology, there are two cornerstones: the active participation of the patient and absolute sobriety as a result. If someone offers "dose control," "treatment without the knowledge," or any other "help" - this person cannot be called a doctor, no matter how he introduces himself.

The provision on absolute sobriety is not even a doctor's suggestion, but a requirement of a sick person! It is unlikely that anyone had heard that the patient persuaded the doctor to cure him not forever, but only temporarily. Nobody wants a recurrence of the disease. Usually, doctors are forced to avert their eyes and speak old words like the world: "medicine is not omnipotent …", "we are doing everything possible …" "I do not give guarantees, but I will try to help you …" In these dialogues, patients are perplexed: "How so? I need an absolute result! Is it really impossible to achieve complete deliverance?"

A sick person is actively seeking help, requires it. He will go through all the experts, read a lot of literature, he will look for everything that can help him. Arguing like this: "Well, okay, I'm an alcoholic, leave me alone," "maybe I'm really sick, maybe I need to pause," the person contradicts himself.

Recognizing himself sick, the alcoholic transfers the situation from moral and ethical to medical. Therefore, the question: "And what if I am an alcoholic, I can't drink already?" By itself, this is meaningless. The doctor is not a lawyer and does not answer legal questions. Is it possible to cough? Can't you walk with a toothache? But what if sometimes, on holidays, I have a rash and a fever? What isn't it possible?

All in all, as opposed to other types of sickness, the cure starts and ends with you!

Chapter 2:

"I Am Addicted" is a Decision

Indeed, it turns out that a person ultimately makes a diagnosis of "dependence" on his own. This is no longer a diagnosis, but a decision made forever.

In our life, we make not so many such decisions. These are such decisions as: choosing a religion, choosing a bride (or groom), choosing a profession, choosing a place of residence. I am an alcoholic; this is the fifth decision from this series. Here, on the fingers of one hand and counted to five ...

Such decisions can only be made by responsible people. That is why alcoholism is extremely interested in ensuring that its slaves never grow up. Often you have to see "teenagers" at 50, 60, and even 70 years old. In the conversation, they show some coquetry, look away, turn the conversation to another topic, or, conversely, gaining false courage, shut up, as if in interrogation, sternly looking to the side. Such a patient all the time wants to end the conversation with the famous phrase of a teenage bully: "I will not be scolded anymore!"

In fact, the person who made this decision has a certificate "I have matured to old age." Unfortunately, not everyone succeeded.

All of these have something in common:

Firstly, these are decisions that are made without logic, without evidence, without theorizing, without reasoning, without analyzing the past. Indeed, no one at the wedding asks the question: "What do you love for?" Such reasoning in such conditions seems tactless and meaningless.

In such cases, the answer "Yes" is yes, and the answer "No, maybe yes" is regarded as the answer "No." The main idea is that if evidence is needed, then there is doubt. You cannot prove to yourself: I am an alcoholic. Now you will prove it to yourself, and then just as convincingly prove yourself the opposite. This means that all intelligence will be aimed at refuting evidence when it will be beneficial for the disease. An alcoholic is a person who can pervert any logic. There is only one way out - there is no logic. No evidence is needed; there will be no rebuttal.

In no case should you stop drinking because "everything is bad." This is all bad now; then everything will not be so bad, and then completely good. Hundreds of times, I had to see people who sat down and said: "That's it! I lost my job, family, and health. I need to stop drinking!" It seems convincing; the person has arguments. But, a month or two passes, and he finds work, after six months it seems that his health has recovered, and there the family appeared. And then the most terrible begins - he begins to drink again.

You can't give up for the sake of the family, for the sake of children, for the sake of work - this is blackmail. Such decisions are made for their own sake without conditions. At the same time, if discussions about heredity and references to psychoanalysis begin, it means that there was no solution. This condition is unstable.

A conversation on this topic often begins with a description of the past. Sometimes the doctor becomes the initiator of these memories. You can understand the doctors - he wants to collect an anamnesis to assess the stage of the disease. But, unfortunately, many patients perceive such issues as an occasion to "confession." The "criminal during interrogation" behavior model begins to work: you need to admit to the little things in order to hide the main thing.

As a rule, a conversation starts "from afar":

- Five years ago, I received a doctor's order for 1 year and did not drink 1 year and two months...

So I want to "continue":

- So, maybe you are not an alcoholic since you received more than the doctor planned?

The decision is forever taken on the basis of the here and now principle. It does not matter, by and large, how the disease developed - slowly or quickly, paroxysmally or smoothly. What happened before the day you recognized yourself as a patient should no longer affect the direction of thought, as it may affect the recovery period.

Secondly, such decisions are made without taking into account the opinions of others. No one can know what to do in such a situation. In making such a decision, the person declares: "I do not know how to, I know how I need to." No matter how close the interlocutor is, authoritative, in such matters, everyone warrants

28

for himself. There are no right or wrong in such decisions.

One has to see how, after talking with the doctor, the patient ends up in a company where some professor claims that sometimes it is necessary to drink. Say, alcohol washes away plaques on the vessels, relieves stress, and, in general, drunkenness is our national trait. Is it necessary to explain what decision the alcoholic will make after this conversation, whose arguments will seem more convincing to him. Do not even argue with such a professor. He speaks correctly. He needs to drink - well, let him drink. And if some prominent actor or minister will recommend me who to marry, which church to go to, whom to work with? Such "advice" can only be taken as a stupid joke. This does not mean that my interlocutor is stupid or a person whose opinion is not worth listening to. This is simply not his business. One train went left, the other right. Which of the drivers is wrong? Yes, no one, they go in different directions. No need to teach anyone to live. And let no one teach you this either. Each has its own fate, its own choice.

If an alcoholic begins to hate drunkards, he is annoyed by the advertisement of alcohol; he fights against alcoholism around the world - this means that the topic itself is not indifferent to him. He is still there in the affected area. This is a huge risk to him. After all, hatred is the sister of envy.

Thirdly, such decisions always force a change in lifestyle. It is important to understand that sobriety is not just dryness. This is a state of mind, a stage in a person's life. The stage, which not everyone reaches, just as not all were soldiers, students, not everyone marries. Absolutely everyone stops drinking, but the happy ones succeed in life.

It always happens, he remains the same as he was, nothing happens. If a person decided to become military personnel, then a lot will have to be changed. Remaining "in the soul" of civilian service, you will turn service into torture; you cannot resign as a general.

Also, in sobriety, preserving all the luggage and not acquiring new, a person remains the same deeply sick, easily vulnerable. One of my patients, realizing this, said: "I simulated sobriety for two years."

Many understand that it is necessary to change and make a typical mistake, starting to change their lifestyle. They declare: "I will be good. I'm giving up drinking, smoking; I'll be faithful to my wife and go in for sports!" It seems that everything is right, but nothing will come of it. Such a person will have to test willpower for strength, and, as we have said, the willpower of an alcoholic is not in his hands. It seems otherwise, but it is not always clear who controls a change to drinking habits.

You Need to Start by Changing Priorities

Initially, a person changes priorities, as determined by a goal. Then the way of thinking changes, and the way of life changes by itself. As in the example of the military: at the beginning, the man had a goal - to become a general. He took the oath, learned the charter, serves. For this, the boots are not heavy, and the uniform is beautiful, and the service is not a burden. In a few years, it will not be clear to him why not everyone is in service. What seems difficult and incomprehensible to civilians will be easy and taken for granted. The lifestyle is like a large barge, which was built and loaded for more than one year, and even ten. Standing on the deck, it is very easy to turn such a ship. Everything is simpler - you need to move the anchor, and then it itself will turn with the current.

Willpower and courage will be needed only to make a decision: "I need Sobriety!" With this in mind, a person gradually begins to think differently, and then he does not recognize himself that he has changed so much.

It is very typical that, stepping into sobriety, filled with the desire to preserve it, at all costs, many are preparing themselves to be provoked. Whole phrases are prepared (sometimes with obscene language), which can be used to refuse drinking. It's funny, but it turns out that these "bombs" are not needed. The patients themselves say: "I suggested a couple of times, I refused, and no one insisted ..." In any case, when there is a goal, these problems go away by themselves. You just have to be firm. This is one of the first steps to treating your sick mind.

Chapter 3:

Five Stages to the Bottom

So, we have discussed a strategy. Unfortunately, as a rule, a "quit drinking" conversation starts from the end - with tactics. At the very beginning of the conversation with the doctor, patients and others literally throw themselves with questions: "What can you offer?", "What is it called?" "How much does it cost?" Important, very important questions, but they should be asked second. First, you need to understand what the patient wants to get. It is impossible to discuss what to go on if you have not decided yet where. At the same time, if there is a point on the map, you will get there. How? It does not matter! Though walking, whatever. The main thing - you know where. If a person really made a decision, then everything will become easier and clearer.

Five steps lead us to such decisions. This is denial, anger, bargaining, despondency, and reconciliation. These five stages are a universal algorithm for solving all problems that cannot be solved by willpower.

For example, we walk along the road and see an unfamiliar beast. The first thing we will experience is the denial: There is no problem, the beast is peaceful; it does not threaten us - just pay no attention. Most of the tasks we solve in this way - we do not pay attention.

But, if we see that the beast begins to threaten us, growls, behaves aggressively, we also begin to behave aggressively - we get angry, stamp our feet, raise a stone. Everyone reacts differently. Very often, going to the door, and trying to turn the handle, we pull it, if it does not immediately open. This method is also quite effective in most cases.

But, if this also did not help, then the intellect turns on, and we begin to bargain. In the case of the beast, we will offer him friendship, sausage, and try to distract him. We need a compromise or full benefit.

Having tried all the methods and have achieved nothing, we will begin to show the beast that we ourselves are afraid of it. Sometimes it works.

And only if this did not help, we will understand that we need to make a choice: either go and let them bite or change the methods.

It is important that reconciliation is not a solution, it is a choice, but a choice only between two paths. There will be no third. We tried to find the third, while we bargained, but did not find.

The same steps can be traced in the decision: "I am an alcoholic."

It all starts, as a rule, with denial. It seems to man, and to others that nothing terrible is happening. Events are perceived as strange but funny. Often relatives are even offended by the assumption of alcoholism by a family member. Patients themselves, as a rule, starting to explain their behavior, build phrases starting with the words "just ..." "I just went over it a bit" "It just happened." At this stage, people turn to numerous psychologists, psychotherapists, astrologers, and other specialists and non-specialists, with only one goal - to find a simple explanation of what is happening. Explanations are found - stresses, politics, stars, etc. A person can be in denial for quite some time.

In general, you need to understand that in alcoholism, the terms are long. This beast does not want to immediately kill the victim. Dates are not calculated in months, or even years. These are decades, lives, and generations.

Most often, denial lasts 10-15 years, then a person gets angry. In this state, the problem becomes apparent. This does not mean drunken anger, but what happens to a patient in a sober state. Coming out of another binge, such people begin to blame everyone for what is happening. They are determined to change the situation once and for all, but as a result, they see the "normal" use of alcohol. Under the "normal" refers to the use without consequences. There is no question of controlling the dose: "I will drink as much as I want!" The main thing is that without consequences. To understand that this will never happen, this person cannot say this to me, and therefore begins to look for the guilty.

Man is angry at himself. But anger cannot be accepted on oneself, and therefore it spreads to others. It's a shame that during this explosion, anger spills over to loved ones. The pattern is also obvious - whoever is closer got the most.

As a rule, a person does not stay in anger for long. Anger quickly tires, though. However, some like it. Such people can stay in it for several decades, fighting their shadow. Causing harm to themselves and others, they seek out everything bad in everyone seeing the enemy.

Sooner or later, a person begins to understand that there is some problem, but he is still not ready to make a decision. In this case, the third begins, and the most terrible phase is bargaining. This stage is really the worst, if only because it is the longest. Most alcoholics die, continuing to bargain, and failing to go further. Bargaining is what doctors most often see.

At this stage, patients determine their condition using lexical evasions: "I'm probably an alcoholic, but not yet chronic" or "I'm a household drunk."

The bargaining goes in everything, not only in definition. Consumption patterns are being built that are constantly changing (only three glasses, only in the evening, only on holidays). The schemes collapse like sandcastles, but, returning to their anger, the patient begins to bargain again for the next scheme. At the same time, intelligence works at breakneck speed, bringing only new losses.

I would like to tell you more about the losses. The fact is that during a bargain, a person can lose and often loses everything. Absolutely everything: money, health, love, faith, respect. This bargaining is meaningless since it is useless to bargain with a creature devoid of morality. Alcoholism is a creature from another world; there, in the underworld, there are no concepts of good or evil. Haggling with addiction is as stupid as reading sermons to mosquitoes about biting badly. The disease definitely decided to suck you to the last drop, and no arguments will convince her. An alcoholic plays infernal roulette, loses, but continues to bet. Helpful logic helps him lose everything: "If I lost 10 times, then I will definitely win in the 11th!"

On this path, a person has a dangerous feeling that he is still doing something. To the question:

40

"How are you?" He replies: "So far, bad. Recently, there was binge again, but I'm working on the problem." He is sure that he lost the battle, but not the war. The knowledge that interests him relates either to the use of technologies (the so-called drinking culture), in which he is "helped" by the advertisement and the "experience" of friends. Or a search for excuses: why am I drinking wrong? Here, unfortunately, a huge "bear service" is provided by psychologists, astrologers, and other consultants who start a conversation with the phrase "you are not an alcoholic ..." How often do you see people using intelligence to build an alcoholic alibi: "I have eustress," "crisis like Martin Eden's," "the hard work that makes everyone drink," not to list all. The science-like nature of these explanations is striking.

But, nevertheless, alcoholism continues to collect its terrible harvest. The patient will give everything, even what he hid "for a rainy day." He will give himself, having come to this satanic temple, and sacrificing all.

The worst thing is that spiritual values are lost. That for which a person could stop drinking. It is very typical that an alcoholic tries to stop drinking for his family. When he states this, he does not lie! He really loves his wife, children. For a while, he was in a dry pause; as a rule, this worked wildly, feeling guilty. It seems that everything worked out. But, after a few months, when the will of the disease prevails, the failure is repeated again. Trying to explain to himself what happened, the patient comes to the conclusion: "I have a bad family." For the sake of this family, he will never stop drinking.

No matter how many times he later creates a family, each time he will have to find flaws in it in order to drink.

If you stop drinking for work, it turns out that the profession is uninteresting. There will be nothing left; all life will be lived in vain. It turns out that the only way out is to get drunk.

In no case should you stop drinking for something else but you! Having to spoil the most valuable for excuses will be painful and incomprehensible. It has already been mentioned that such decisions are made only for themselves, for yourself, because you have come to such a conviction!

Trading daily for years, the patient begins to acquire the "stigma" of the craft. Just as a shoemaker can be recognized by the stoop, a teacher by voice, and a policeman by sight, and the trader has characteristic features.

Firstly, in trade, there is no faith. You can't take the proceeds in an envelope; you need to count. If they brought a box, let them open it. In the same way, an alcoholic never believes in 100 percent and never in anything. If he is shown to a person who has stopped drinking and has not been drinking for 5 years, the "merchant" will draw conclusions for himself: either he drinks, but imperceptibly, or did not drink at all, or will soon get drunk. It is hard to believe that there is treatment, help if you do not believe in the result.

Secondly, there is always a third way in trade. From the very beginning, trading was the art of compromise. If the merchant is not able to solve the problem, not as it should, but as it can, he will not receive benefits. Is it good or bad? It's good for a merchant, bad for an alcoholic - because his life is the subject of bargaining. And the "customer" is a creature more powerful than him. A creature that has already destroyed more than one billion people. But the search for the third way takes the patient's mind completely. Even in a conversation on this subject, it is very difficult for the patient to answer "Yes" or "No." Everything revolves around "probably," "maybe," "suppose," "what if suddenly ..."

Thirdly, the merchant firmly believes in a pagan miracle. Surely someday the necessary deal will turn up, I will behave correctly, and then the size of the gain will be such that I have enough for the rest of my life. But for this, you need to observe the rituals: "don't take money from your running capital," "say the right words," etc. If we are talking about the seller, this is just funny.

This phenomenon takes a completely different turn in alcoholics. These patients are absolutely sincerely convinced that there are "Naltrexone" pills "for binges" (not for alcoholism). They are constantly looking for some additives, herbs, sorcerers. Confidence that if you search "as it should" - you will find something that no one knows about takes on the form of super-valuable ideas.

By plunging into bargaining more and more, a person becomes confident that he has become a specialist. The most typical phrase: "Doctor, I don't need to tell anything. I know everything!" The naivety of judgment is not visible to the patient, since he really went a long way, very tired, but moved in a circle. So he didn't leave anywhere, he lost everything without finding anything. How can a person learn something new if he is sure that he knows everything?! In order to go on a journey, a traveler must assume that he has not been everywhere. In the same way, an alcoholic will be able to understand something only if he understands that he does not understand anything.

During bargaining, there are situations of temporary dryness. This is not sobriety, namely, dryness, because the decision is still far away. This is a situation when a person has already lost almost everything, but health is still left. There is nothing to take from him, but he can earn. And then alcoholism seemed to let him go. A person suddenly decides that he will not drink for a year or two, and does not drink. It works, and makes friends, a family appears. As a rule, everyone believes that he will never drink again. Although, in a conversation on this subject, the alcoholic himself suggests that sooner or later, he can still drink. Of course, not like before, but soon the vow will end. The word can and is the pitfall that this ship will crash about. He cannot help but drink. After all, the rope on the neck remained! And when you "walk up your sides," you will be pulled again, and you

will have to come and leave everything again –
another vicious circle!

Few manage to complete the bargain in life. Most patients die, continuing to bargain, but if all the same, the bargaining is over, the patient proceeds to the most unsightly situation - to despondency.

Being discouraged, the patient already agrees that he is an alcoholic; he does not argue, does not bargain, does not seek contradictions in words. He understands that he is drunk, but believes that this should be done carefully. There is no doubt that alcoholism turned out to be stronger, but it is reliable that at least he will be allowed to die without pain. A person is no longer looking for a good job, although, as a rule, he continues to work in order to drink. He is not trying to restore relations with loved ones; he even eschews them, realizing how bad it is. All judgments, intentions, fantasies are built, taking into account how he will drink at this time. Whether, after drinking, will be able to finish the job, or is it better not to start it. There is no doubt that he will drink. Such people are not aggressive, although others show concern for them, experiencing biological disgust. They reckon with a drunken bully and despise the homeless, although, from a person in gloom, the harm is much less. It would be logical to show compassion for him, but not understanding how this could happen, people feel fear. Fear that generates aggression.

Be that as it may, but despondency is a step forward.

Only after these circles of hell does a person come to reconciliation. To the situation of choosing from two possible options.

There are no barriers at these five stages. Easily out of gloom a person can go to bargain or even show anger. Angry about it, make sure of denial. As a rule, after all, bargaining is the most frequent manifestation, because, exactly, the soul rolls into it every time.

Those who are fortunate enough to make a choice in the direction of freedom are changing so much that it is rather worth talking about rebirth. Even if such a person has breakdowns, he no longer hides them but analyzes them. He is extremely interested in everything that can help him; he is trying to be crystal honest with himself. He wants, and sooner or later, he can be responsible for himself.

But making a choice is not easy. Bargaining instilled a desire to find the "third option," and therefore, the situation "go left - go right" does not suit. An alcoholic is looking for a "door in stone." He is confident that if you are a little trickier, you will still be able to deceive, slip through. Such people say: "Yes, alcoholism is a terrible evil. This is a plague that has already claimed many of my friends. This is grief. But I still try to go around the edge, not to fly off this turn, especially since I have really important reasons for drinking."

Paradoxically, the one who made the choice "I will drink, drink and die" has a better chance than the one who made no choice. It so happens that, having come to the conclusion: "a bottle is a ladder to heaven," a person is still horrified and changes his mind, but, pay attention, he already had at least some solution. It is much worse when a drowning man cannot grasp one edge of an ice hole. This means only one thing - he will continue to sink.

What is the "Bottom," and What is the Ultimate Way Out?

All who have received sobriety described the time when they experienced a sense of bottom. The bottom from which they managed to push off. There is such a feeling, but it's descriptions always look very strange. On the one hand, you need to feel it, but at the same time, they always warn: "Look, don't miss it! There is no bottom in the swamp!" People around are waiting for the bottom to come and ask: "What are the signs that a person has already reached a dead end?" There are no such signs. This feeling is mental; it is without sensations, without objective indicators.

When a person graduates from school, he is overwhelmed with a feeling: "This stage is over, now everything will be different!" But there were no sensations. There was no pain in the forearm, no temperature, no rash. What clinical analysis will show that a person decided to marry, become a poet, or go to another country?

It turns out that there is a sense of the bottom, but you won't run into the bottom with your heels. Rather head, or where a person's soul is? It is very difficult to determine: what is the bottom of an alcoholic and if he is already or not at the bottom.

How many times had to see patients who, due to frostbite, which happened while drunk, had to amputate their fingers. How many people committed terrible crimes while intoxicated. Sometimes an alcoholic even partially realizes that he is doing poorly and consciously goes for it, believing that "after this, I will definitely quit drinking." But, some time passes, and everything returns again. Although it happens that insignificant losses (loss of telephone, quarrel in the family, loss of work) suddenly cause a person to feel horror and an understanding of the bottom. Sometimes relatives tell each other about such cases and make the wrong conclusion: "He will drink until he crashes the car. I'd rather break it!" It doesn't mean at all that if someone stops drinking after a divorce, the other drunkards will do the same. There is simply no universal recommendation. Thousands of people lost cars, families.

One gets the impression that a person draws this line for himself. But, having drawn, it no longer erases.

The bottom is really a state of mind. And he understood, then changed his mind, again proved something and returned. But what's important is that the bottom is just a choice, not a decision. There are those who say so to themselves: "I have long reached the bottom. I was knocked from below, and I went on."

The feeling that I am already at the bottom is a feeling of complete emptiness, an understanding of absolute loss. In fact, this is a recognition of defeat, not a temporary failure, but complete impotence.

Realizing that he has reached the bottom, a person recognizes himself not as a beggar, but as a debtor. One patient described this condition as follows: "I had a family where they were afraid of me, there was work that they did not respect me, there were a house and some things, but they did not bring me joy or peace. It seemed to me that I had all this for rent; in fact, all this did not belong to me..."

Recognizing this, a person gets the opportunity to change something, at least he has a choice. But recognition is not easy. Pride does not allow us to let fears go. It seems that impotence cannot be recognized, we must fight on, and everyone says: "you must fight, you must hold on."

The bottom is a refusal to fight.

Paradoxical as it may sound, it is precisely the rejection of the struggle that allows a person to change direction. One alcoholic said that he had a feeling that he had been trying for a long time to open the door until he realized that it was opening inside. You just had to stop pushing it. In fact, the refusal of attempts to change something by his will saves the alcoholic.

Many, trying to help an alcoholic, try to bring him to the bottom, indicating to him his loss. This is quite logical, but we forget that we are faced with a paradoxical disease that distorts the psyche. It is extremely rare to convince a patient that he has "everything as bad." Patients, like in a frying pan, try to get out, build endless arguments and excuses, and then, often, tired of making excuses, suddenly say: "Well, since everything is so bad, therefore, nothing more needs to be done."

Talk about this irritates not only the patient but also the one who is trying to lead them. As a rule, these losses are joint: not only did the patient lose several years of his life, but his family members also suffered. Therefore, the conversation takes place on increased emotional tones and is very reminiscent of the accusation. As already mentioned, a person with alcoholism is "ready" for the charges. He begins to "explain everything" - others insist - excuses are becoming more and more elaborate and aggressive. This "walking in a circle," as a rule, ends with a banal scandal that does not lead to anything but unnecessary stress.

As practice shows, the patient himself must come to this concept. Until a person independently experiences a feeling of complete loss, there is no point in convincing him. Therefore, it is better if, during a conversation, others do not talk about their losses, but about him. No need to make assumptions "if you did not drink." You do not know what would have happened in reality if the alcoholic hadn't drunk, and you would be "caught" on this logical mistake - be prepared. Tell us what really happened. After all, a lot has already been lost. Speaking about yourself, describe not losses, but your state of mind. What did you experience when it all happened? This will help you understand yourself.

Do not demand the result immediately. It often happens that a person must think, remember what they were told, compare, evaluate. And, sometimes, it is possible to draw a conclusion.

Chapter 4:

The Identity of the Alcoholic

The personality of an alcoholic is full of contradictions. An alcoholic is a teenager with an old-fashioned outlook on life, this is a professional deceiver who is quick to spend, this is a complete egoist who does not love himself, this is the eternal "soul of the company", who is forever alone, this is a hero you cannot rely on, finally, this is a person who is not afraid of death because he is afraid of life. The list of these paradoxes can go on for a long time.

The thing is that in the personality of an alcoholic, there are two individuals. No matter how it sounds crazy, but it is. In general, we have already said that alcoholism is precisely insanity.

The first personality is different for everyone, with different childhoods, different intellectual abilities, different worldviews, etc. But the second personality is the same for all patients. This is extremely important to understand because often, you have to see how a patient, sometimes together with "specialists," begins to delve into his childhood, social environment, and education to look for the causes of alcoholism. As a rule, these searches end only with the creation of the next alcoholic alibi with hopeless conclusions. Ah, here it is! I had the wrong upbringing, but it's already impossible to go back and change something. Therefore, starting is not worth anything.

The fact is that the very second person could have developed with anyone. People with different religions, places of residence, and the history of generations. She did not grow up with the patient, did not study, did not earn respect in society. This is really a parasite that has settled in this soul and now forces itself to feed.

The doctor knows the second person very well. In no case should it be perceived as a manifestation of individuality.

The second person may seem primitive, but only at first glance. First, to manipulate the situation, the opinions of not only the patient but also those around him, the intellect of the patient himself will be involved. Secondly, she knows how to wait. She has different ideas about time. It doesn't matter, week, month, year, or decade. This demon is immortal; he has nowhere to hurry; he is sure that he will wait for his own. Thirdly, what is obvious to us is not at all true in that painfully distorted logic. Strength can be used as weakness; values can become insignificant, or altered altogether.

There is a statement that alcoholism is a disease for the smart and strong-willed. This is partly true, but not in the sense that all smart and strong-willed people should become alcoholics, but in the sense that the patient will have to use his mind and will to serve his master.

The situation is really paradoxical. Many are surprised: "How could such a strong person get into such bondage?" The answer is simple: the second person never orders directly. It always stands, as it were, from the back, sprouts in the first, and dissolves in it. A person begins to perceive those desires, thoughts, and sensations as their own. He constantly faces a problem: why did I want one thing, and then did it differently? We used to find simple explanations for everything, it's easier, and therefore they can be found.

Often you have to see the superficial judgments of alcoholics, in some strange way combined with a love of resonance, theorizing. Obviously, the discussion of the topic is so emotionally intense and painful that I want to either skip it or take the conversation aside. The most typical answer to the question: "Do you need sobriety?" Is: "Do you want to hem me?" It seems that if you ask the question: "Why do you answer the question with a question?" You will get the answer: "Why do you need this?" As a rule, after the second or third phrase, you have to hear: "Well, that's it! In short! You can't do anything! You don't have anything concrete!" Sometimes a long story follows about archetypes, enzymes, historical references. And when you ask: "Why are you telling all this to me?" You see genuine surprise: "How, didn't you understand anything?"

This behavior is common as alcoholics are very touchy people who are ready to offend anyone. But the fact that the alcoholic is very touchy is not immediately clear. Firstly, the nature of resentment is not always clear, sometimes there are resentments for some nightmarish tricks of drunken friends, and sometimes the patient will be offended by the remark of a neighbor. Secondly, even if you do not touch such a person, he will still find a reason for resentment. He will be offended even by what is shown on TV. One gets the impression that he just needs to pick up some insults in order to fall into a state of emotional madness. Such a slight vulnerability is noticeable even to the patients themselves; they conclude that they are "thinly sensitive" natures, they are surprised at the "thick-skinned" nature of those around them.

The most revealing manifestation of resentment is the constant willingness to experience "righteous anger." Patients love to be angry, just feel the need for it. In anger, they always come to the same conclusion: "With such a life, how not to drink?!"

It is a paradox that with such easy vulnerability, patients show a surprising indifference to those they love. Even to themselves. Less and less, they are affected by events in the family. They gradually do not care what they are wearing.

Attitude to their health, as a rule, is polar: on the one hand, they like to talk about blood pressure, stomach, kidneys, which they get naughty with all the time. On the other hand, it costs them nothing to go out to the street naked, drink to stupor. Coming out of binge, many patients begin to be frantically treated, take drugs for the liver, go to gyms, and become tempered. One gets the impression that they are very cherishing of themselves, but during the next binge, the body will get such an injury that all these therapeutic measures will be useless.

A description of the paradoxes of the psyche of an alcoholic can be carried on for a very long time, but all this does not explain what is happening. The clearest picture is obtained if we assume that this person is truly two-faced. And he does not give himself this report. His intentions seem to be good, but since he did not determine the goal, it is with these intentions that the road to hell will be paved.

For many patients, sobriety began with the understanding that there was me and someone else. I had heard one patient say: "I once realized that if I want to drink, then this is NOT I want. From that day, I began to stop drinking..."

Tunnel Vision

The term "tunnel vision" in medicine refers to ophthalmic problems in which the peripheral region of the retina suffers for one reason or another, and therefore a person's peripheral vision worsens or is completely absent. Such conditions are found, for example, with retinopathy pigmentosa (Usher syndrome).

However, in psychology, this term has taken root quite firmly, where, of course, something else is meant. In this case, tunnel vision is understood as a person's concentration on any one idea, sensation, or memory, which makes it difficult to cover the whole situation. In narcology, this concept is also often mentioned, but, as a rule, in the context of the desire to drink alcohol. Most of the references to this phrase produce the same simple sentence: "tunnel vision - when all thoughts are directly or indirectly concentrated on use."

One way or another, but the phenomenon of tunnel vision is described in sufficient detail by psychologists studying the problem of dependence. And, analyzing these observations, one has to speak more about "tunnel vision" rather than "tunnel thinking," or even "tunnel psyche."

Let's analyze this phenomenon in order, namely: emotions, memory, and thinking.

Emotions

In people who have a dependency on themselves, in the assessment of surrounding events, in the field of feelings and emotions, very often have to see a certain narrowness. In the description of emotions, as a rule, there are few adjectives. A person does not even try to search for synonyms for a more detailed description of feelings. Some experts call this emotional impoverishment. But I want to emphasize that the intensity of emotions can be quite high. The "unethical" description of feelings is often understood by others, and by the person himself, as a sign of "simplicity": "...what nurses! I am a specific person; they said - well, that means excellent!"

The question: "What do you like best?" Often causes such patients surprise. Sometimes the answer is philosophical reactions: "How can this be compared?" And more often just annoyance. If you analyze the speech of such a person, you will notice a certain set of standard ratings that these people use. It is noteworthy that in this set, there are practically no gradations: two or three definitions for the concept of "good," a little more for the concept of "bad," and a few for the concept of "nothing." "How good" is generally not rated.

Memory

The volume of memories is often limited. We will not classify palimpsests here - the lack of memories of what happened during the binge. In a sober state, as a rule, memory begins to "come back." People begin to remember some details of their life for quite long periods, but, nevertheless, these memories are fragmented. The memories of being on vacation, on a business trip, are usually associated with drinking. Sometimes these are memories of some vivid emotional experiences. Unfortunately, most memories are associated with particularly vivid experiences and do not spread over time. A person remembers the moment of experience, but poorly restores the picture before and after. Often these are negative experiences, which sometimes creates a person's full sense of the "nightmare" of his past life. Some people realize that it is not so bad. But they remember, for some reason, it's bad. And these memories then do not go away for a long time.

Thinking

This is an assessment of the situation. It has long been noticed that patients with alcoholism are categorical in their judgments. Sometimes this is even interpreted as a sign of infantilization, but, apparently, this is not entirely true. In the case of infantile judgment, a person can easily experience strong sensory experience, attachment to a person, object, or phenomenon. Teenagers tend to create idols in the "ideality" of which they are confident. However, in this case, people begin to collect information about this phenomenon, willingly discuss it, and tend to communicate with other "fans." At these meetings, the amount of knowledge about the object is taken into account during a social assessment, etc. The main condition of such communities is the invariability of the assessment.

In the case of an alcoholic, a person makes a hasty conclusion, tends to give an unambiguous definition, and move away from the discussion. Patients insist that they provide the "essence" of the method. Outlined the "most important thing." Details, as a rule, are of no interest to anyone. One of the most common questions in response to the sentence: "Do you need sobriety" is: "What is this?" For a person familiar with the problem, such a question seems generally incomprehensible. But experts know that the patient expects to hear: "Yes, this is a binder (chemical protection, coding), etc." After that, the question will be direct, like a shot: "How much?" Well, and so on...

It is clear that such a dialogue does not lead to a detailed study of the issue. Often, after an offer to go to a rehabilitation program, patients respond: "This is not mine!" That's all. It is proposed to end this conversation.

Analysis

Patients with alcoholism are not prone to analysis. This does not mean that they do not like to talk about the "topic." On the contrary, some talkativeness is a fairly common phenomenon. As a rule, these conversations are in the nature of a certain resonance, similar to schizophrenic, but without a broken logic. It's difficult for patients to talk about a specific issue for a long time. The theme easily gets off to another. It seems that the person has already made all the conclusions, and he is not interested in this anymore.

Often I had to see how someone tried to convince an alcoholic using the "on the contrary" method. He began to describe the benefits of sobriety: "Stop drinking, buy a car, make a career, create a family." It was supposed to take the next step: "But for this, you need to do something, first make a decision!" But, alas, no one reached the next step, meeting the answer: "I don't need a car, I have work, and women, enough!"

Decision-Making

In patients with alcoholism, decisions are made impulsively. There is no desire or opportunity to make a decision deliberately, carefully.

Patients are prone to simple solutions. Decision-making is "torn" in time: "I will do it now, and then I will get it" As a rule, there is no planning of the implementation process itself. Cases seem either extremely simple or unworkable. Starting something, a person does not imply painstaking activity. Very often, you have to hear from patients who have heard a lecture on addiction: "So! This is all good, but what am I to do now! "

The answer is supposed: "Go to the next office, there you will be quickly treated, then go to the cashier, pay, bring the card to me with a check."

Such an "algorithm" seems most acceptable to patients. The question: "And then what?" is not supposed, and if asked, then there is an answer to it: "And then everything will be fine!" The mistake of reasoning is that an alcoholic who just got out of use does not know, cannot answer himself myself to the question: "What is good?"

People cannot get what they wanted because they did not know what they wanted. It causes frustration, despair, anger, and - the next breakdown.

There may perhaps be only one recommendation: to learn to see what is underfoot. To do this, you do not have to "run," but "walk." Do not give ratings, but if you give, then take into account that your estimates can be clearly overstated or underestimated. Live one day, and try to do everything possible in that one day, but nothing more. Do not give promises of results, promise actions to achieve results.

Keep in mind that there is something else in this world that you could not see due to the fact that your eyes are still wearing blinders.

Chapter 5:

The Way Out

So, we got to the main question: "What to do?"

For all the correctness, this question is meaningless. It is clear what to do - do not drink! Many people fall for this particular trick. Endlessly answering the questions: "What to do?" And "Who is to blame?" These people wander in the dark, walk in circles, looking for something under their feet, and cannot find because they don't know what it looks like.

The question should be posed differently: "How?" How not to drink to a person affected by the disease that guides his actions?

Most people answer right away: "How! Do not drink, and that's it!" Let's nevertheless move away from superficial judgments, stop looking at the situation primitively, and begin to understand: "It's simple, but not easy." You can't recommend an alcoholic to show his willpower: "You are a man!" "You are a strong woman!" In no case do not offer values for the motive: "You have a family!", "You have a public position!" Do not set conditions: "Throw away the drinks - buy a summer house."

This decision should be made just like that! We have already said that there should be no logic.

And now, if this decision is made, then the most important thing begins. Such a person has a lot of serious and difficult, but interesting work. The job is to understand - where you are and where you are not already. You need to understand yourself, to understand which manifestations were yours and which have already come from the side of the disease.

It is imperative to understand that talking about a cure is unacceptable. Dependence, having infiltrated the soul, never leaves it. But this does not mean that there are no people who quit drinking. There are such people, even quite a lot, but these are not former alcoholics, but people who have learned not to obey addiction.

It will be a question of a skill that is painstakingly given, not in one session, you should not count on it. The skill that only one who learns by himself receives. No, and there will never be tablets with the skill or obtaining the skill "by proxy." And finally, the skill that anyone can gain. There is no such thing as a person studying, studying and not learning.

If nothing came of it, it means that he has not started anything yet. In addition, I repeat - it is simple, but not easy.

The most important recommendation is: "Start talking on this subject!"

Many, hearing this are perplexed. Apparently, our brain is so designed that "thought is born in the mouth." Never can a person understand what is happening to him until he calls it a word. Named by the name of demons, a person manages to get rid of their influence. I emphasize influences, and not from the thoughts themselves. Such thoughts will surely appear more than once in this sick soul.

Very often, you hear: "Make sure that there is no traction!"

To be extremely precise, the patient feels the "craving" or compulsive attraction immediately before the breakdown. This is a condition that covers the entire sphere of desires, and, as a rule, then it is no longer possible to avoid consumption. In other words: traction is a state when there is no choice.

If a person has experienced cravings, it means that it is too late. But until the craving appears, nothing is felt. It turns out that to the question: "How are you?" The patients answer: "No craving!" Of course not! If there was a craving, we would have already noticed. You can do something so that there is no traction. This is the result that must be obtained.

No, and there has never been a pill, an injection, or any other way to control desires. It is scary to imagine what would happen if someone could change the desires of another person at their discretion. The request: "remove the craving" consists precisely in withdrawing one desire, leaving all the others.

Often you hear that "flushing" the liver, cleansing the body of "toxins" and extorting "stress," a person may lose traction. As a rule, these "miracles" are offered by specialists from the field of resuscitation, toxicology, or even people who have nothing to do with medicine. If you think about this proposal, it may turn out that if the offender rinses the liver, then he will become a righteous person? Unlikely.

Very often, all these manipulations are used by a sick consciousness as a bargaining chip.

78

Yes, of course, the internal organs of the alcoholic were very much affected, and, of course, droppers and preparations for the liver are indicated for such patients. But to believe that this will eliminate cravings is naive.

There are drugs that cause alcohol intolerance. This therapy is called sensitization. Opinions about these methods are quite mixed. Some specialists and patients who have stopped drinking alcohol consider that such methods are unacceptable, that the risk of death in the event of a breakdown in therapy is too great, and not worth the result that the patient receives. Some, on the contrary, insist that otherwise, patients cannot cope and offer to regularly receive such medical care.

First, I would like to talk more about such methods. This therapy is not new today, and, like any other business, has become rumored and speculated.

To start with, these drugs do not eliminate the desire to drink but make it impossible. None of these substances are centrally acting, psychotropic, tranquilizing, or antipsychotic.

Secondly, the insult of people declaring: "how so, I drank and did not die!" is not quite clear. And what would be better if he died? So, he was a good doctor, experienced, and guessed that you would drink?

The cruelty of people convincing "friends" who received such medical assistance that they say "you can drink, you won't die!" I immediately want to ask: "and if he dies, do you agree to be responsible for the death of a friend?" Yes, there is no 100% in medicine, someone survived two and three reactions to alcohol, and someone may become disabled from the first glass.

In any case, everyone should understand correctly - such manipulations are only a safety net for the first time. You can't file the ability to swim; there are no injections with knowledge of a foreign language. If I did the procedure - well done, well done, this is a solution worthy of respect. But this is only the beginning. Consider giving crutches. Not forever, but only for a year. If you learn to walk with crutches, then maybe you yourself will let go at some point. But if you haven't done anything all year to learn to maintain sobriety, then you'll lose it.

Unfortunately, the most typical situation is the policy of "hard-drinking in a year." You see, a patient who was given a medical treatment a year ago. Now the term has expired, and he has gone into a bar. To the question: "what did you do while you didn't drink?" The answer: "I worked, I worked very hard, seven days a week, twelve months a year." If you ask: "What did you do to maintain sobriety?" You will receive in response: "I was not drawn. I did not have any cravings at all. Let's try medical treatment again for a year, and in a year, we will meet again."

It is important to understand that this is not a result. Even wives are sometimes offended. What a wonderful life! All year to endure a person "on the platoon," afraid that soon there will be a binge, count the days, and when this happens, experience horror and disgust!

Sobriety is a valuable thing, given in good hands. It's like getting married. If you marry once a year, no one will say that you are a family man.

Often people ask: "And for how long is it better to quit?" This is not an easy question. Some people think that it is better to start with short terms: half a year, a year. And there, if everything worked out, you can increase it to three, five years. Many experts are convinced that if you managed to persuade the patient to do the manipulation for the maximum time, then start with five years. As an argument, the provision is given that in one year, you will not have time to understand anything.

The conclusion is clear that if a person did the procedure for three years, and after a year broke, then repeated procedures do not make sense for more than a year.

Perhaps the correct recommendation is to let the patient decide for himself what time is clear to him, what period he can imagine. It is significant that when a patient requires a binder for 25 years, they usually ask him: "Can you imagine what you will be like in 25 years?" Usually, people answer: "What are you, for me three years is infinity!"

Figuratively speaking, leaving the fog does not need jumping. Simply put your foot in a visible place. It is much nicer to see the person who made the medical protection for six months, at the end of the term, has come and consults on whether he can now do the procedure for a year. It is important that after the period of action of the drug, there was no breakdown. Climbing the stairs, the main thing is not to slide down; you can walk slowly, but not back down.

But, even after I did the procedure, it is necessary to begin the most important thing - to acquire the skill that was already mentioned.

Treatment should begin on the first day of sobriety, and not stop.

School of Sobriety - A Step to Acquiring the Ability Not to Drink

If maintaining sobriety is a skill, then obviously there are schools where you can get it? Yes, there are such "schools." This book will only talk about a few of them, not because the rest are bad, but because this story can be endless.

We have already discussed that the most important method is the need to speak on this topic without intoxication. These conversations should be conducted in a confidential atmosphere since their main task is to achieve absolute, crystal honesty in relation to oneself. People with whom I can be so frank should inspire confidence in me. Not reverence or submission, but trust. I must be sure that they will never use what I said against me.

Such conversations should be perceived as medical manipulation, a doctor's recommendation. They should not be delayed for external reasons. It's like a wound dressing. If the doctor said - once every two days, then we will bandage once every two days. Not knowing why, without thinking, why so often. This recommendation should be followed even if the patient went on a business trip or is tired.

I don't want to talk about this topic, or rather, I don't want to speak! It will not work right away; conversations will seem absurd, meaningless. At first, it may seem that there is no benefit from them. We agreed - this is a skill. It is necessary to continue. Not immediately, but to succeed in any case.

The easiest way to conduct such conversations in the family. Many of the patients were lucky; they managed to save their families. Family members are people, which you trust; there is no sense in hiding something from them, especially disease.

This must be done at least once a week. Actually, the more often, the better. The fact is that the aggravation of dependence takes about one to two weeks, and therefore, if we try to understand ourselves in a month, we can skip it.

This procedure should go into the family ritual: every week, on some pre-selected day (usually before the weekend, although there are no clear recommendations), in the family, we should talk about how we are doing on this front. As a rule, these conversations are conducted between spouses, but I had to see how the patient opened to adult children, a friend on a fishing trip, or in a bathhouse.

Rule one

During the conversation, only one topic is discussed - the disease. These sentences are not accepted: "I don't want to talk about this topic!" "Enough to shame me already!" "There are more important topics!" There is no more important topic for the patient. If you are sick, then there is nothing to be ashamed of. We want to show compassion - so let us do it! Often it turns out like this: they started from the main thing, and then somehow got lost on events in the world, a summer residence, with relatives. Therefore, we immediately agree the next hour, for example, from 21:00 to 22:00 - only about the disease, about yourself, then about relatives.

Rule two

During the conversation, you need to describe not events but feelings. Unfortunately, we often conclude that the events of our lives are directly related to sensations. For example, in response to the question: "How was your day?" You hear: "I woke up, went to work, returned home, had dinner, watched TV, and went to bed." This is a well-written police report. Now it is clear where and when I was, but what I felt at this time is completely not clear. Description of the day may look like this: "I woke up in a good mood, spring, birds outside the window, I wanted to go to work. I walked joyfully. When I arrived, I suddenly found out that today is Thursday, and I thought Friday, tomorrow is a day off! Somehow I was immediately upset; I didn't want to do anything; I worked "on the machine." But after lunch, I developed nausea. I already have to go home, but I still thought something else needed to be done. Now I'm sitting and thinking that I need to call someone I don't know." Please note - there were no unusual events, but how many sensations! This is what we need to talk about.

I would like to draw attention to the fact that some people try to use the terms to describe feelings: depression, frustration, etc. Believe me, it is more useful to say those words that you understand. No need to be shy. If a person says: "Covered, flattened, dragged ..." it is much more effective than a cutesy "depression" without understanding what it means.

Rule three

You need to talk to someone. It is unlikely that a person is able to be extremely frank with the wall. In order to understand if you are not lying to yourself, you need to look into the eyes of the person you are talking to.

The result of such a conversation should be an understanding of where your illness is now. If "everything is good," there is no illness, then something has been hidden, once again lied to yourself, tried to embellish, not to disturb. So, the disease is from the back, it simply is not visible, but it is very much alive. This is a very dangerous situation, you don't see it, and so it's easier for it to order you.

How often do you have to see a patient whose wife left yesterday, he has not been at work for a week, probably fired, there is a mess in the apartment, and in response to the question: "How are you?" He replies: "Everything is fine! Do not worry!" Now, if I heard: "Doctor, I have a problem!" I would become less worried.

Unfortunately, such conversations in the family are not always obtained. Not because the family is bad, but because the thoughts and feelings associated with the disease look so bad that sometimes they feel sorry for loved ones. It's scary that they will be afraid of what they hear. One patient told me this case: "My wife went to see my relatives, she's delayed, and I'm worried. This is normal. And, suddenly, I thought, what if she had an accident? And then, can you imagine, a wave of positive emotions swept over me. I am alone at home; I have grief, I can drink! No one will blame me!" He said that even a cold sweat had come out. "What a crazy person I am, if the trauma or even death of my beloved wife makes me think of a drink!" It's clear what not to immediately decide to tell your loved one. But you will still need to tell. Otherwise, these worms will then turn into snakes.

For such cases, there are places where patients can gather and talk among themselves. These are the so-called rehabilitation programs. In my opinion, the term is not very successful. Firstly, because the word "rehabilitation" in many countries has had a political connotation for a long time, and, secondly, because the word "program" resembles working with a computer more than with a soul. But that's my personal opinion. And the term itself has taken root, and now it's probably not worth changing it.

The main condition of these programs is anonymity. Not secrecy or mystery, namely anonymity, as a condition of security, since none of those present knows who the other is. That is why, on such groups, one can say what bothers, without fear of evaluation.

The most universally recognized program can be called the program "12 steps," Alcoholics Anonymous. The main advantage of this community is that it was created not by academics but by alcoholics. This is not the fruit of scientific research, but the experience. The experience of people who did what helped. The program is old in the good sense of the word, and it has already been tested enough and has established itself as a way by which more than one person got the result. Today, "12 steps" is a worldwide phenomenon that does not have clear signs of a national mentality. The program is quite versatile and well debugged. We'll talk more about it later, but for now, just know that there is such a place, and not one.

In addition to this, there are other programs. In many cities, there are many places where you can get this help.

In further addition, there are people burdened with an oath, who promised never to tell anyone. Conversation with such people can also take place in a confidential setting. Sometimes you hear a misunderstanding of the term medical confidentiality. Say, the doctors swore that they would not say anything to the patient. Also, all over the world, there is such a specialty - a psychologist. These are people without medical education, but they, nevertheless, also declare anonymity in helping, and promise to keep a secret.

Finally, there are people burdened with a very ancient oath. I am talking about ministers of the church. In all traditional religions, the secret of confession is accepted. Alcoholism is understood as instilling into the soul of a demon. It is believed that a drunk person is obsessed with demons, and a sober person who has experienced such a thing is possessed with demons. The demon is cunning, assumes different guises, does not order, but constantly tempts hides and lies. Most of all, the demon is afraid of the truth, and he is indestructible. There is only one way out: every day all through life to follow the purity of thoughts and intentions, comparing them with the will of the Highest.

I would like to draw attention to the fact that there are no contradictions between medicine and the traditional ideas of mankind about God. In fact, we are saying the same thing; only the words are different.

Chapter 6:

Clinic of Exacerbation of Dependence

I would like to separately describe the exacerbation of dependence as a clinical manifestation of the disease. Knowing how this condition develops provides us with the ability to protect against hard drinking.

Dependence - What is it?

Dependence is a chronic disease and therefore manifested by exacerbations. By exacerbation, we will understand the complex of symptoms that precede binge, because, after the first glass, it becomes clear to wish for this "pain" more and more.

An exacerbation of addiction is a psychiatric condition, and therefore it is unlikely that a blood test or x-ray will help us here. These are manifestations of pathological thoughts, sensations, and desires. Manifestations are not explicit, so you should not prioritize the situation, saying, "I don't feel like drinking!" Not everything is so obvious in this state. You need to be patient for painstaking work.

As a rule, exacerbations are cyclical; that is, they are repeated at certain intervals - once a month, or three months. Seasonal exacerbations are very typical. Aggravation to a sharp change in the weather. In fact, any fairly severe psychological trauma can trigger an exacerbation.

It is important to understand that the aggravation goes on for some time. The most typical period is one or two weeks. This is important because understanding this means we have time to react to prevent the condition from becoming irreversible after drinking.

The leading symptom of exacerbation is anhedonia, a specific sensation of a lack of sensations. It is extremely difficult to describe this condition since an ordinary person almost never experiences it. There are no such words in the language to clearly, succinctly, and clearly, name what is happening in the soul of an alcoholic these days. Patients themselves describe this sensation as "lack of spring ...", "lack of celebration ...". Patients complain that "... everything has become somehow fresh, ordinary, routine ...", "Nothing pleases, and everything is tiring." Some even try to get carried away with something, start repairs, start some kind of business, projects, but, alas. Even what usually gave joy, turned on, now it passes somehow "by itself," "mechanically." Everything around seems somehow inferior, does not touch us, does not give a full perception. One of my patients very figuratively described this condition: "I'm like a spider in a jar. The world is like behind glass. I see everything, but I can't touch it." As a rule, there is no feeling that "everything is bad." Everything is not bad and not good - just nothing. Everything seems to be there, but something is missing. "It feels like I've bitten off, but not swallowed," said someone. There is no indifference, a person wants to get something, but even to clearly state that he cannot.

Sometimes it begins to seem that the patient knows exactly what he needs: "I'll finish the car painting," "I'll buy a phone," "I'll finish the job," and then ... But as soon as he begins to think, "what then?" confusion appears in his eyes and discouragement.

Non-alcoholics sometimes experience something similar against a background of an infectious disease, or extreme fatigue. The differences are that in people without addiction, this condition does not last long. As a rule, a day or two, or even hours. Here, however, anhedonia can last up to a month. This state in itself becomes a holistic phenomenon that requires registration on the part of consciousness.

Depression - What is it?

Depression is a feeling of underestimating one's actions, merit, and qualities. Underestimations are not necessarily human. It seems to the patient that the events are also not going the way he would like, complaining that "they do not fully realize themselves," "their talents are not in demand," "with their intelligence and ability to work, they deserve much more." How much a person is right in such judgments is a difficult question. Indeed, many alcoholics are extremely able-bodied and talented people. The soreness of judgments lies in the conclusions: such a person does not decide that something needs to be changed, but simply begins to accumulate resentment. Such conversations are very reminiscent of ordinary envy, but unlike the white envy, "You are great, I'll try so too!" Or the black envy, "You are better than me, so I will destroy you!", The alcoholic has some kind of gray envy. Such a person argues as follows: "Everything succeeds, and only my fate is this. Nobody appreciates me." The result is not an achievement of the goal (in good or bad ways), but resentment itself, hopelessness.

Ideas of Relationships

These are expressed in the fact that the patient begins to think that others have changed their attitude towards him. As a rule, there is no feeling that "everything is against me." There is a feeling that "everyone does not give a damn about me...", a feeling of complete indifference of the whole world to you. Most of all, it hurts the feeling that family members have become "indifferent" to you. The last word in quotation marks is because this is usually not the case. Objectively, the attitude of others does not change, but the patient perceives the change in relations very clearly, although he cannot, at times, explain to himself why this is caused. The wife of one of their patients told:

- A week before the breakdown, he begins to ask: "Do you love me?" Well, of course, I love, so many years already together. The question is romantic, but how did it end? Hard-drinking for two weeks.

Relationships deteriorate not only at home but also at work. Even on the street, at random encounters, it seems to a person that they did not pay enough attention to him. Here are the words of one of the patients:

- On such days, it starts to seem to me that all the passersby's are pushing me, they don't see where I am going, I, like an invisible person, all look "through me." I go to the store; the saleswoman doesn't see me, chatting with someone as if I were not there.

Many people describe that on such days, food becomes tasteless, unsalted. The patient begins to smoke more or changes the grade of tobacco to a stronger one. Watching a movie or a book does not give a full sense, it appears that "everything became worse, not like before."

The patient is increasingly comprehended with "disappointment."

- So, I was thinking, I'll take this position, buy this thing for myself, get acquainted with this person! Bought, borrowed, met, now sitting and thinking, so what? There is no joy in owning anything!

Against this background, pathological thoughts begin to appear. These thoughts are formed incorrectly, and therefore their occurrence, course, and resolution follow painful laws. Most normal human thoughts arise in response to a situation, are accompanied by emotions, and require logic to complete. For example, a person wants to buy an expensive thing, but there is not enough money. This is sad, unpleasant, and here an emotion has appeared. So, you need to work harder, maybe borrow money, or refuse, if you don't so much want. Logic processed the situation; the thought was gone.

In a state of exacerbation, everything happens a little differently. In the beginning, an emotion appears, by itself, due to internal, painful mechanisms. Consciousness is trying to attach this emotion to some situation, and there is a surrogate "reason." Then the logic appears, but this tool does not work, since there is no beginning, and therefore there will be no end. The patient begins to return to this thought again and again, and cannot find a solution in any way. Patients often call this condition, "I drive."

- Well, I found out that a neighbor went on vacation to an expensive resort. I don't want to go to the sea, I don't know how to swim, but I go and think, why am I going to the country for a month, and he is at sea for two weeks?

From the outside, such thoughts look disgusting. You'll not tell everyone. And those who are told evaluate this see it as boring.

The boredom of an alcoholic is a fairly common symptom. Many perceive this as a character trait with age-related changes, but the cycle is more characteristic of the disease. A person can walk with a normal emotional background for several months, and then begins to get bored. The environment is annoying. The patient himself often also understands what causes irritation, and therefore simply hides his feelings, tries to get rid of them, guided by the old rule: "Just don't think about it!" Unfortunately, it's easier said than done. How not to think if you decide not to think?

Efficiency against the background of these experiences, as a rule, does not decrease, but rather increases. The patient begins to take on more and more stress, trying to overcome anhedonia, having achieved at least some extreme sensation, for example, a feeling of extreme fatigue. Fatigue – the feeling is simple, understandable, requires no explanation, no evaluation.

Helpful logic is connected: after all, I will get what I wanted, I will prove to everyone who I am!

It is important to understand that this happens without the knowledge of the patient's personality. Direct questions: "Why do you need all this?" "What do you want to prove?" Cause confusion in the patient: "Well, isn't that obvious?" "But how else?"

In fact, a person "goes to pieces," works a lot, sleeps a little, does not eat regularly, and then, as a conclusion, he gets into a binge against a luxurious alcoholic alibi: "I have had a lot of work; lately, I'm very tired!"

The insidiousness of the disease lies in the fact that you think you do not want to drink all this time. It often happens that family members, friends see changes in the patient's condition, pay attention to his mood, behavior. They remember that the last time it ended in failure and trying to help the patient, they ask: "Do you want something to drink?" In response, they usually receive a negatively emotional response: "No! I have no desire to drink. I do not feel traction. Leave me alone with such questions!" After the beginning of the binge, everyone is offended by the insincerity of the person: "We felt that things were amiss. They asked him. Why lied!"

By and large, the alcoholic did not lie; that is, he was honest with others, but he was lying to himself.

Not everything is so simple in diagnosing this condition. Firstly, indeed, the patient himself cannot feel the deterioration. He can notice it, understand it, but there are no sensations in the body. Secondly, not everyone has a picture that looks exactly as described. All people are different, in some patients, some signs prevail, in others - others. Thirdly, even periodicity is not always logical. I had to see people whose aggravation developed so rapidly that they could not even notice it. Such people claim:

- "I understand what you are talking about, but it happens for me in a day or two. It seemed like everything was fine yesterday, and suddenly, I wake up with longing, all day in vain, the next day disappointment, irritability, and now, I'm ready for a breakdown!"

Sometimes patients, on the contrary, say the following:

- Yes, that's exactly the way it is, but I have already had it for a year. Fluctuations are, but small. Out of binge, I immediately go into exacerbation, endure, then again a breakdown. A few days after the hangovers seem to be normal, and again envy, anger.

What recommendations can be given to people who nevertheless decided not to obey the disease, and not bring the aggravation to failure?

The most important thing these days is to sit down and analyze what is really happening to you. For this, we need to talk on this topic. The bad news is that when the exacerbation has already begun, it is extremely difficult to start such a conversation. That is why the topic should always be open. If a person has the skill of such conversations, if such an opportunity has already been worked out at a time when the state is stable, then it will be easier for him to start such an analysis even when everything is bad.

The second recommendation is to reduce the load. As a rule, on such days, he does five to six hours at a time, and even more. He is all in the hassle of repairing, a car, documents, work, family, country house; he just has no time to think about himself. A remark from others or specialists: "You have looked bad lately, don't want to pause?" Meets a condescending smile and an answer like: "What else should I look like when there are so many things to do?" Indeed, even distribute what are the most important things now, and then move to more difficult tasks.

A rule of cases is proposed:

- "I do no more than three things at the same time. When I finish one of them, I can take up the next."

- If the case does not end within a week, I stop and put it off till later.

This rule immediately causes a storm of indignation: "It's easy for you to say!" You must remember that this is not a friendly wish but a medical recommendation. Failure to do so can lead to a breakdown, and then there will be neither money nor time, and the family is unlikely to be happy.

In some cases, it is necessary to prescribe sedatives to patients. To date, psychiatrists have a fairly large arsenal of tools that give an equalization of the emotional background and do not have significant side effects. It is clear that the appointment of such substances can only be after consultation with an experienced doctor who has the skills to work with drug and alcohol addicts. If a person suffers from addiction, he can get addicted to almost any substance that changes consciousness. Although, for some reason, it seems to the patient himself that "he will never become a drug addict ..." Therefore, we can only talk about prescribing drugs for a short period of time - one to two weeks, with long breaks in courses. If everything goes well, and the patient is sobriety for more than a year, as a rule.

Some patients on such days successfully use drugs of disulfiram (Esperal, Teturam, Lidevin), or cyanamide. You need to understand, as already mentioned, that these substances do not eliminate the desire to drink, and in no way affect the emotional background. They only give intolerance to alcohol, which is hedged for a while.

One way or another, but every exacerbation lived without a breakdown, is another coin in the box of sobriety. With each such victory, a man moves away from a nightmare longer and longer. Further, it will be easier, just as the wound is healed, and subsequent exacerbations will go through large periods of time and will flow more easily.

Do your best, use only a positive and drug-free experience to get this result.

Chapter 7:

The Workable Program of "Alcoholics Anonymous"

Starting the description of the "12 Steps" program, I must say that I am not a representative, leader, or authority of the community of Alcoholics Anonymous (AA). However, it would be a huge omission not to describe this phenomenon in a book on the treatment of addiction.

Unfortunately, in practice, one often encounters the fact that patients have some fragmentary, and often erroneous, information about the program. What is only worth mentioning is that they say there are some "Intimate alcoholics," "Secret alcoholics," or even "Autonomous alcoholics." As a rule, patients have the opinion that this is either a religious sect, or a club of moderately consuming people, or some kind of elite clinic for actors and artists.

One of AA's traditions says that their activities are based on the attractiveness of ideas, and not on propaganda. This chapter will describe how the author himself understands these ideas without claiming to be evaluated.

From a clinical point of view, this program gives quite significant results. Throughout the world, it is the "12 steps" that are considered the most civilized way to solve the problem. One gets the impression that "this horse" has not only pulled out, but is it right or wrong from a scientific point of view? As a practicing doctor, I try not to ask such questions, especially since the opinion of scientists about the effectiveness of such programs is very diverse. Sometimes, diametrically opposite.

The main thing that needs to be understood is that "12 steps" is a program of spiritual growth. This is not clinical detoxification, not employment, not communication training, but a place where a person can understand himself. Other members of the community can help him in this, but everything that he does, or that he misses, will be done by him. No one will lead him or assume his responsibility. Indeed, this is the concept of freedom: do what you want, do not bother anyone and bear responsibility for what you have done.

Depending on the translation, the steps in different publications are somewhat different, but the main idea is the same everywhere.

The first step: they recognized their impotence before alcohol, came to the conclusion that they were not controlling their lives.

Many, having heard this at the AA meeting, immediately experienced a negative denial: "I thought I could gain strength here, but they are powerless!" The idea is that, only by recognizing powerlessness, a person can refuse to continue trying to do what he always did.

Powerlessness is not weakness. Weakness is partial; it humiliates a person, impotence is absolute, it magnifies. The recognition of powerlessness is an adult solution, only knowing what you am capable of, you can develop, otherwise, you will have to continue to test the world for strength, finding out what you still cannot do. Powerlessness is a great thing since it makes the prohibition unnecessary. A person does not need to forbid himself to lay down on the rails in front of the train, as he recognizes his powerlessness in front of the locomotive. If he sees this as a weakness, he will have to forbid himself such actions each time until he deceives himself and still tries to commit an insane act. The recognition of powerlessness is a victory over temptation, not a struggle that draws into excitement and anger, but an opportunity to pass by. In fact, the recognition of complete powerlessness will allow a person to escape the curse of Sisyphus.

Another step in the program is considered by many as the cornerstone, "castle stone." It consists in the fact that we have entrusted our will to a higher power, as we understood it.

I often had to see people who, after these words, literally jumped up and ran away from the meeting, believing that they had gotten to some sectarian sermon. Many have explained decently that I am an atheist, an agnostic, and, in general, if I want to talk about God, I will go to church. Firstly, this is a later step; not everyone started with it; in addition, some, starting with the search for God, immediately became religious fanatics. There is a position in the community: "First come to the group, then come to yourself, and then to God." In any case, the Alcoholics Anonymous steps are not a sect, and everything is done in order not to become a sect. There will be no sermons; for this, you really need to go to the temple.

An alcoholic is a mentally ill person, and therefore it is quite natural that this is a program of spiritual growth.

Alcoholics Anonymous is not a religious program: they do not recommend mentioning the name of God at a meeting - everyone has his own ideas. There are people for whom the Higher Power generally does not appear in the form of that God, which is customary to be mentioned in traditional faiths. People believe in Universal Justice, in the Wisdom of Nature, in the expediency of existence. It does not matter. The important thing is that these people have a sense of life, not earthly, momentary, which can be considered differently depending on the situation or mood, but comprehensive, not depending on the circumstances and opinions of others.

Many said that before this step, there was a feeling that you were trying to get out of the ice pit, but the walls were slippery, and no matter how fast you walked with your feet, you would still go down. And only after they managed to tackle something unshakable, the situation began to change for real.

Another important step involves trying to convey the meaning of our ideas to other alcoholics - the final one. Many began their sobriety with the "fight against alcohol." They literally attacked a drunken neighbor, dragged a relative by the hand of a group, or a doctor, met an addict, and then spent all their time and money on her treatment. As a rule, this "battle" ended with the breakdown of the agitator himself. It was bad for the patient and terrible for his wards. Imagine what thoughts appeared in people who seemed to start to believe, and suddenly, saw him drunk.

After 3-4 years of sobriety, a person has a natural desire to share the experience. Not to lead, not to save, not to control the fate of others, but to share experiences. In fact, this step is important for a beginner; he must understand that no one owes anything to anyone here. These people want you to come. They are glad: there is someone to tell about themselves, and you can be grateful to them for telling you this.

There is the prayer of Alcoholics Anonymous. Program members themselves do not claim authorship. I often heard "offended" people who found the "historical truth" and claimed that the author of these words was someone else, and you, as they say, ascribe them to yourself, or incorrectly indicate the author. I would not be surprised if I find out that these words were inscribed on the walls of Babylon, and since then, people have been repeating them.

These words are: God give me reason and peace of mind to accept what I can't change, the courage to change what I can, and the wisdom to distinguish one from the other.

Chapter 8:

Co-dependency

This chapter is worthy of a separate book, but I will try to describe at least a few pages what is happening with the people who surround the alcoholic. This condition is called co-dependence, and this is not just a term, it is a diagnosis of the disease. This disease, like dependence, follows its own laws and has common features in all patients, regardless of the individual carrier of the disease. This is extremely important to understand because the anosognosia of the co-dependent - the non-recognition of one's painful condition - is so common that it is considered one of the manifestations of the disease.

Usual stereotypes tell us that the co-dependent is a woman, the wife of an alcoholic, a person with limited intelligence ("... only a fool can live with that ..."). Imagination depicts us as a weak, depressed personality, not paying attention to their own appearance, in whose eyes there was a feeling of fear. Alas, this is not entirely true. Of course, there are such cases, but not in most. Such people are striking; the seal of their grief is obvious.

It's quite clear for a specialist that a well-dressed woman, the head of a large organization, fully dedicated to the cause, strong and tough, is simply afraid to come home and, therefore, literally drowns herself in work. When a man takes responsibility for what happens to his wife, trying to heroically "solve her problem," the expression on his face appears like that of a fighter, "burdened with a special mission." Anything can be said about this, but it would never occur to anyone to show compassion for him, recognizing that he is unhappy.

However, this is nothing but different faces of the same disease. One way or another, but these are people who cannot afford to be happy.

Many co-dependents are persistently interested in everything that can be done, but not for themselves, but for the alcoholic patient, not recognizing that they themselves also need help, and no less than an alcoholic. Sometimes, in a conversation, they even admit that they have been living in a strange way lately and that something needs to be changed, but "this is not the main thing," "... now, we will deal with his problem; then we'll talk." How it reminds the statement of the drinker ", this is not the case."

Often you have to see the genuine indignation of wives who are offered help: "... you doctor should not be worried about that!" "Do your thing. Your task is to make sure that he does not drink, and somehow I myself will figure it out!"

Burdened with a load of information, these people begin to believe that "salvation is near," and they no longer want to hear anything. The deception is that they see salvation not for themselves, but for the patient. And your problem should melt like snow in the spring.

The essence of co-dependence is that these people are in a state of chronic fear. This is the native fear of primacy - the fear of the misunderstood. The co-dependent cannot understand the mindset of the alcoholic, and therefore is afraid. Fear is a disgusting feeling, the fear is humiliating, and therefore, the consciousness is trying to "cover" it with something. A person begins to experience sensations that must exceed this ugly feeling. As a rule, this is a feeling of hyper-demand. It is hyper-, since only severe, obviously exceeding the norm sensations are able to hide this fear under themselves. A set of similar experiences also includes aggression, perfectionism, sacrifice, theorizing, and doom, many faces of this demon.

The identity of the co-dependent seems no less controversial than the personality of the alcoholic. On the one hand, these people really want to "get to the bottom of the essence," but they do not intend to listen to anyone, since "everyone already knows." They are ready to give "everything if only he would not drink," but this should happen somehow quickly, in one session, without painstaking work. They understand that the disease is incurable, but insist on compulsory treatment. In fact, one has to see paradoxically formed relationships. This is a kind of aggressive adoration, people who are ready for the death of loved ones out of "love" for them.

Very often, in a conversation with co-dependents, one has to explain the patient's refusal to implant Esperal. The doctor explains that the patient does not intend to stop drinking alcohol, does not believe that the drug will work, but nevertheless, if he starts to use it during therapy, he may be in intensive care, become disabled or die. In response, you can hear scary words, like:

- So let him die! If he becomes disabled, I will look after him, all the same; I can't live!

- If everything is so bad, it's possible to disperse it in a civilized way.

- No! How could he be without me - completely die!

- "But you were just ready to bury him." Do it yourself!

There is only one way to deal with a demon - call it by name. You need to start with the fact that a person simply admits, but he feels a sense of fear that he can't cope with, because he will never understand the patient.

Do not try to understand the alcoholic; God forbid you to understand this. This painfully distorted world, where the same images can be presented in different forms, can only be understood by one who has been there. Trying to sew his logic to what is happening, the co-dependent begins to look for the guilty. Such are: friends, work, time, vodka producers, government, and the co-dependent themselves are guilty. There is hatred towards these people and phenomena. A sizzling feeling that kills not from whom it is directed, but from whom it emanates. The wives of alcoholics are eagerly involved in the fight against "drunkenness," with the advertising of alcohol, with drug treatment doctors who are "unable to turn their husbands from drinking." At the same time, the assumption that the problem inside is in the soul of the alcoholic himself does not suit. Often, summing up the story of the co-dependent, they want to ask: "So who is he? Monster or sick?" Unfortunately, one often hears the following: "What kind of alcoholic is he?" He is a bastard!"

Help for Do-dependents

In short, the recommendation for the co-dependent is to accept the situation as follows:

He is sick - you are staff. Personnel not eligible for empathy. Empathy and compassion are not the same thing. In fact, these are mutually exclusive concepts.

Firstly, the staff are people who are obviously healthy. Sick staff will not be able to provide assistance. Therefore, the first task of the co-dependent is to admit that they have a problem. Not only with an alcoholic, but also with them as something happens that is not subject to their desire, not explainable by logic, and not depending on their will. Only then will you be able to turn the problem into a task and begin to understand what needs to be done. In any case, one should not give money to a drunk, under no circumstances, one should not bring alcohol, one cannot justify a drunk, call work, and say that he is sick. You can't change your plans, depending on the state of the alcoholic. Do not serve binges. Start worrying about sobriety.

Secondly, the staff are people who know what to do, and if they don't know, they don't do anything. Very often, I hear from family members of an alcoholic: "We are at a loss; we do not know what to do." As a rule, these are the same people who make every effort to get a wonderful result: "so that I woke up and find he did not drink." It turns out some violently active despair. Panic is prohibited for staff. Always starting a business, you need to know in which case you will need to stop if your actions are ineffective.

When you start explaining this as co-dependent, you often have to see indignation: "Are you proposing to leave everything as it is?" No, I propose to stop doing what was done before! Yes, you need to increase the distance. Emotionally, and not necessarily geographically. I had to see wives who divorced, separated, remarried, and now come from the other end of the city to their first husband in order to "go out for a beer," "clean up the apartment," "call a doctor."

The increase in distance should by no means be perceived as a betrayal. This is a medical evacuation from the lesion. There are situations in which you are powerless; you cannot help. Being in such a place means increasing the number of victims. Let there be people who are saved and ready to meet you. It is important.

The co-dependent should have a "plan B." The plan of retreat, the plan of salvation. This plan should be thought out to the smallest detail. You cannot scare an alcoholic. If a wife said a hundred times that she would leave, but did not leave, this would not work. "I'll leave" - this means where, when, what I'll take with me, everything thought out. This is the condition for implementation.

Such a plan is necessary for the patient - this is one of the conditions for motivation, and for the most dependent - only such a plan will save from panic. We must know for sure: what will we do if we realize that we can't do anything.

Remember that even increasing the distance, moving away from the nightmare, you will still carry within you the seed of your disease. You will be addicted to addiction. For a long time, the word "alcoholic" will speak in your soul, like an explosion of dynamite. You will still want to sacrifice yourself, feeling the seal of the curse on you. Unfortunately, you have to see how a woman leaves her husband an alcoholic and remarries another alcoholic. Escaping their circle of this nightmare is not easy, but possible. First, you need to make a decision that "I also have a problem that will need to be addressed."

Start living well; for you, this is a medical recommendation, not a wish.

The Invisible Part of the Disease

What the wife, parents take for the disease, in reality, is only her half.

The most difficult thing in treating drug addiction and alcoholism is the treatment of the parents or spouse of the addict or alcoholic. I admit that this sounds unexpected, but it really is. They are sincerely mistaken, believing that their son is seriously ill. No! In fact, the whole family is seriously ill! And the addict's parents are no less sick than himself, even if they don't want to admit it. Some of them believe that addiction is such a disease in which a person uses intoxicants to experience intoxication, high, as a result of which certain biochemical changes occur in his body, which is called a physical dependence syndrome. They believe that the disease is shots and bottles; these are muddy eyes and attempts to take scores with life; these are terrible breakdowns, comas, and overdoses. In these states, the most terrible things are done. These conditions make the strongest and most severe impression on relatives and friends. Perhaps this is why some parents believe that the entire clinic of the addiction syndrome is exhausted by such manifestations. And this is really part of the disease, but only very small. Some parents, taking a small part for the whole illness, are deceived in what is happening. Based on such false premises, they treat their son accordingly - with drugs, detoxification procedures, "cleansing," biologically active additives - and are disappointed in the treatment eventually.

And if you look closely? More inquisitive parents will notice that both without intoxication and without "breaking" their son/spouse's behavior has been significantly changed. He is unstable, quick-tempered, depressed. He cannot work normally; his thoughts are far away, outside the family. And even if he remembers his parents, he's only to "pump out" more money from them, to dress him, to feed him, to take care of him. At the first opportunity, he recalls drugs (alcohol) and rather does not stop thinking about them at all. He is deceitful, quirky, cunning, cruel and capable of exerting tremendous willpower in order to get the next dose. All these are manifestations of the syndrome of mental dependence. Parents of a drug addict (alcoholic), who were able to recognize psychological dependence by persuading, take their son to an appointment with a psychotherapist. But such treatment sometimes gives only short-term results, which disappoint parents even more. So what is missing for success?

But the fact is that a large addiction syndrome, consisting of syndromes of physical and psychological dependence, is only half the disease. And the other half is what I call parental dependence syndrome. Even when it comes to marital relations, the wife, in such cases, assumes the role of the mother in relation to her husband. More often, this condition is denoted by the term - co-dependence. This is just what you did not treat, something that does not allow you to achieve lasting and lasting success.

Alcoholism and drug addiction as a disease is not only the process of stupefying and finding funds for drugs; it is not only the breakdown and suffering of the addict. Almost half the disease consists of the reaction of the parents to the actions and reactions of the sick son, which can be both healthy and painful. If the reaction of the parents is adequate, healthy, correct, then the problem is solved, the son refuses drugs (alcohol). And if the reaction is erroneous or even painful, the problem is aggravated, and the son's disease progresses rapidly.

Since drug addiction is represented by many symptoms, and the parents of a drug addict can react differently but erroneously to each of the symptoms, the syndrome of parental dependence seems to be the most difficult and biggest. And given the fact that co-dependence also precedes alcoholism and drug addiction, is fixed in time and in itself is one of the most important triggers of the disease, then, in my opinion, it weighs up to half the clinical picture of the whole disease in weight, volume, and significance.

I must say that drug addiction, alcoholism - a syndrome of dependence, this is a multi-cause disease. A variety of risk factors or different combinations of such factors can trigger an alcoholic illness. For example, factors such as the weakening of the body by a disease, the consequences of traumatic brain injury, birth injury. This can be the consequence of great stresses, such as military service, hot spots, loss of loved ones. Finally, domestic disorder, the consequences of chronic stress in the family or at work, non-observance of the regime of work and rest, a drinking team at work, a teenage company with a "negative" leader, a genetic predisposition, etc. But the genetic predisposition, like the other of the above risk factors, has never been a significant factor in the formation of the disease!

There is another factor that, by weight, volume, and significance, occupies among the others about 60%, is co-dependence. This is something without which alcoholism and drug addiction will never take place. In independent, healthy parents, children simply cannot get drug addiction. And vice versa. If someone in the family is sick with alcoholism or drug addiction, then other family members must have co-dependence.

Chapter 9:

Lasting Solution for an All-Time Cure

The fact that alcoholism, drug addiction can be regarded as a disease of a person, family, society has already been settled.

Alcoholism. Addiction. Syndrome of chemical dependence. These words, combined with the name of a son or daughter, wife, or husband, cause a cold in the chest, a sinking heart, a chilling fear. How many lives has this disease claimed? How many souls it stole. Someone was able to give up drugs, from alcohol, escape from the strangling embrace of death, and with horror recalls that time as a nightmare. However, more are broken, crushed, destroyed by the disease. Why parents could not help children cope with the disease? Why were the efforts of the wives in vain? How not to repeat their mistakes?

To avoid danger, you need to identify it. But how to see, touch, weigh the chemical dependence? At first glance, it seems that this is an abstract problem. Where is she, the disease? In the head or in the heart? Or maybe the disease has some kind of chemical formula? Perhaps the disease is in a bad company, in friends? Or is it a metabolic change? Illness in drug dealers or in syringes? In beer stalls?

The Monster on Three Legs

Personally, the disease seems to me a monster on three legs. The monster, at first glance invisible, settled in the soul of a person, usually able to stay on only three points of support. And enough to knock out any of the three props to addiction, the syndrome collapses. And if parents and loved ones want this to happen as quickly as possible, less painful for the addict, then it is necessary to deprive the disease of not one, but two points of support at once.

The first support of the disease is in the patient himself. This is a large addiction syndrome, which, in turn, consists of syndromes of physical and mental dependence.

The second pillar of the disease is the sick society in which we live, with its not always healthy way of life, with inhumane, written and unwritten rules and laws, with its sometimes wolfish relations between people. Therefore, alcoholism and drug addiction are classified as social diseases. Their prevalence in society is determined by the direction and activities of social policy.

The third pillar is a sick addict's family. This persistence of parents in upholding their false views and erroneous beliefs, thanks to which the disease found a nest in their family, settled in the soul of their loved one and is rapidly progressing.

To knock out the first support, it is necessary to refer to chapter 5 of this book. If this does not work, then you need to take a medical step, along with the following guidelines, which I shall soon discuss.

In mild cases, this is a one-time intervention, and in advanced cases, it is a long, complex, and expensive procedure consisting of several stages. At the first stage, it is necessary to remove the manifestations of physical dependence, which is performed with a high degree of reliability only in a narcological hospital and is a massive drug intervention. The next step is to stop the psychological dependence. Only a psychotherapist or psychiatrist-narcologist can handle this work. However, this far from exhausts the course of treatment for alcohol addiction syndrome. After the manifestations of physical and mental dependence are removed, after the attraction to psychoactive substances is removed, it is necessary to remove the accompanying changes in the emotional sphere, so that without drugs or alcohol the patient does not suffer and does not suffer, but feels better than in alcoholic or narcotic intoxication. And after the medical stage, the stages of social and psychological rehabilitation will follow.

Thus, the first fulcrum is knocked out. I agree that all this is complicated, cumbersome, and sometimes time-consuming. Is it possible to make it easier and more efficient? Can. It is possible to simplify, reduce and reduce the cost of treatment if a disease simultaneously knocks out the second point of support - change relations in the world around us, in society, or change relations in the family.

Not every parent can allow themselves to change their relationships in the world surrounding a drug addict. To do this, you must be a very rich, strong-willed, or influential person. But, theoretically, such an opportunity exists. For example, parents can change the addict's citizenship, make him a citizen of a country where they treat their citizens with humanity, where, on the one hand, mechanisms for early detection of the disease and forcing treatment are provided, and on the other hand, many social guarantees have been created for the weak and sick. Or another way. If the father or spouse of the addict is a police chief or criminal authority in some "county" city, he can conduct explanatory work among local alcohol sellers, and they will shy away from the addict, like a leper. However, for most persons, this option is unrealistic and is more likely to be in the realm of fantasy.

Thus, there remains one more fulcrum of the disease - the sick family of the addict, the erroneous reaction of parents to the manifestations of the disease. Imagine that for a son to heal; it's enough for parents to change themselves, their views on the problem of family relations, their behavior, and their actions. Yes Yes! Everything is really that simple! The first reaction of parents to such a proposal is emotional. With joy and hope, they immediately agree to comply with all the doctor's recommendations. They solemnly promise and swear that they will do everything that the doctor says, that they will do everything necessary to save their son (spouse). And this attitude is preserved until the recommendations are voiced. Have you seen what happens to a balloon when air is released from it? The same thing happens with the addict's parents (or co-dependent spouses).

The hope of success immediately fades. They, without having tried, refuse to act according to the plan proposed by the doctor. They break their oaths and promises, hiding behind excuses like: "We have all tried this," or "I feel sorry for him," or "I am afraid of him," or "If I don't help all this, then he may perish." And the parents of the drug addict (again!) Are disappointed in the treatment, not only without completing the course but without even starting it. But let me, the statement of the parents that they "have already tried all this" does not hold water. They, of course, tried to do something, but not everything, not so, in other conditions and without the help of a doctor. At the same time, they acted impulsively, inconsistently and did not finish what was begun to the end.

Parents, fearing an aggressive reaction of an addict, should realize that the disease is progressing rapidly and, if you do not follow the recommendations, within subsequent years, they will see a truly bestial appearance of this disease.

Fears that it will be worse or that the son may die are well-founded. But this can happen not because the parents followed the advice of the doctor, but because they began to act very late.

Finally, about what the spell is worth, that "it won't help." How can they know if they have not followed the doctor's recommendations?

In the following concluding chapter, I undertake to prove that saving the life of an alcohol addict is really in the hands of parents and spouses who have overcome co-dependence, overcome the disease in themselves.

Chapter **10**:

Belief in Your Own Strength

The fact is that the parents (spouse) have everything they need to cope with the disease.

Everything in nature is arranged wisely. Spring follows winter, then, summer, and then fall. And there, summer will please us with sunny days. Everything is consistent; everything is logical. There are surprises, yes, there are surprises. But with all the seeming randomness of their manifestations, they are nevertheless predetermined by the whole course of events. The accuracy with which they can be predicted stems from the inviolability of the laws of nature and the universe and is determined by the degree of knowledge, the degree of knowledge of these laws by man.

Medicine, in general, and narcology, in particular, is a fairly accurate science, which means that everything can be measured in it, and any result can be predicted with a greater or lesser error. Alcohol addiction, like other diseases, proceeds according to the laws of human nature, fairly well-known and proven by practice, therefore does not pose a threat to the health of society as a whole in a humane democratic state. Moreover! The level of development of medical knowledge allows you to return to a normal, healthy life, the vast majority of addicts.

"Allows" you to return, but does not return you on its own! The realities of our lives are far from idyllic pictures. Unfortunately, the prognosis of the disease for most addicts in many countries is unfavorable. And this is not happening because specialists are poorly trained and cannot meet the terrible disease fully equipped. On the contrary, I can say that many therapists and psychotherapists dealing with the problem of addiction syndrome have vast experience and invaluable work experience, which allows them to be the best in their field of knowledge.

Then why is the problem of alcohol addiction and dependence so acute in our society? Why is a sufficiently well-studied disease that takes so many young lives and poses a threat to the health of the population of an entire country? But because drug addiction and alcoholism are social diseases. Their prevalence and flow rate are completely predetermined by the direction and measures of social policy. In the group of social diseases, such as tuberculosis, sexually transmitted diseases, and others, in terms of the number of lives claimed and the extent of the damage to health, the dependence syndrome occupies an honorable, undoubtedly, the main place. But with alcohol addiction, there seems to be no phenomenon that posed a threat to the health of the entire population. Hence, it is seen as less a scourge.

But what can we do, even if the state signs its helplessness? The first is to believe in yourself. To believe that your own strength is enough to solve this problem, in order to help your loved one cope with the disease and return to a normal, healthy life. There are many reasons for such an optimistic position. On the one hand, in the hands of parents and spouses are all levers of influence on the patient. Perhaps they were unaware of some of them and did not know how to use them effectively. But believe me, there are many such levers, and they are effective enough to effectively influence the behavior of an addicted family member. On the other hand, a son or daughter, wife or husband, have weaknesses that they know better about than anyone else. Finally, there are specialist doctors with professional knowledge of the disease ready to respond and help in trouble.

And what confronts parents and spouses? A serious illness that settled in the body of a loved one, taking root in the family. The disease is nevertheless predictable, proceeding according to certain laws of human nature, which neither the doctor nor the parents can change. But they can use their knowledge of these laws to help their loved one give up drugs or alcohol forever.

The Desire to Help at the Level of Actions

The fact that the words of the co-dependent sometimes diverge from the deed.

So. On the one hand, a disease that can be treated (and there are many examples), a serious but solvable problem, and on the other hand, a healthy part of the addict's personality, loving and strong parents who are ready to do anything to save their son's life, medical specialists, friends and relatives who are able to respond to a request for help with advice and deed. Who will win? The chances of success in this matter for sober and responsible parents, even in advanced cases, I assess as four to one. There would be a desire to help a loved one.

Parents will say that the desire to save his son was and is, that the desire is very big, but "things are still there." The disease progresses; the situation is aggravated, despite all efforts. What is the matter? Probably the fact is that parents and the doctor differently understand this expression. In the doctor's understanding, "the desire to save an alcohol addict" is not empty and fruitless dreams looking at the ceiling, these are not tears in the pillow. No. This is a clearly defined sequence of actions and steps necessary to solve the problem. This is the ability to take responsibility for everything that happened to this person, for what will happen to him in the future, for everything that happens in the family on his shoulders.

As for the sequence of actions, then everything is simple and does not cause any objections from the parents until it gets to the point. Indeed, success requires the most basic, at first glance, things:

The first one: Loved ones need to collect all available information about the disease, get acquainted with popular literature on this issue. And judging by the fact that you are reading this text, you are already taking the first step to success. But why so far, the parents do not have enough information to solve the problem? The question is rhetorical.

The second thing to do is to find out what kind of training and qualifications a specialist should have that can help solve this problem. Despite the obvious necessity of this step, despite the fact that the individual has been ill for more than one month, and possibly for more than one year, the loved ones of an alcoholic or drug addict, as a rule, have the vaguest idea on this issue. They are surprised to learn that different specialists are required at different stages of treatment, that the treatment process for alcoholism is sometimes always not a one-time procedure. The question is, why so far such information has not been collected? This question to be answered.

The third action: Choose a doctor and, after drawing up a treatment plan, until complete success, clearly and rigorously follow all his recommendations. Can the attending physician of an addict confirm that the parents (spouse) complied with all his recommendations? If so, then the patient will recover. If not, the disease will progress.

The action plan is simple, like three chords, as effective as aspirin, and will not cause objection to any sane person. Then why is it not implemented by the parents of a drug addict? Why do they, with all the desire to help their son in words, do not take sufficiently effective measures to save him at the level of actions? Let me remind you that in the clinic of this disease, and therefore in the behavioral response of parents to its manifestations, everything is pathologically logical, everything is predictable. The reason for this is co-dependence, the syndrome of the parents or spouse of the alcohol addict.

So what kind of specialist will help get rid of a deadly ailment? If we are talking about the treatment of alcoholism or drug addiction, then, of course, the doctor is a psychiatrist-narcologist. And in narcology, the main treatment method is psychotherapy. The most important medical tasks - the formation of the patient's motivation for a sober life, a critical attitude to his condition and illness, an attitude towards sobriety, a desire to solve the problem to the end - are performed only by means of psychotherapy. Acupuncture, laser, devices, and medication are not done. A pill for alcoholism and drug addiction has not yet been invented. Attraction to alcohol and drugs for years is not removed by drugs. There are no such drugs that would last for years. This is also done only psychotherapeutically.

But it happens that a psychiatrist-narcologist specializes in treating emergency conditions in a disease clinic - "breaks off binges," "relieves breakage," and uses limited therapeutic methods in his work. This means that he can help someone in the radical treatment of the disease, but he cannot remove it totally - he needs all the help he can get to be able to do so 100 percent.

Another alcoholic disease is being treated by psychotherapists. Such specialists indicate in advertisements that they treat eczema, psoriasis, neurodermatitis, hypertension, obesity, and alcoholism. But if such a doctor does not have training in the field of narcology, then perhaps he does not know the nuances of alcoholic illness. This means that while he is able to help some, he might not be the best choice for you.

The best results will be with the doctor who presented you with two certificates, a psychiatrist-narcologist and a psychotherapist, and a license for the corresponding type of activity.

The man turned to the reception: "doctor, probably, it is useless to treat me. I've already been treated ten times: hypnosis, coding, acupuncture, laser, injection, filing - for everyone. I grit my teeth for two or three months; I keep myself sober, then I break off." I ask: "And for what type of activity? Have you been presented with a license?" Answers: "I have not seen a license." That is, he was disappointed in the treatment, although still not once. In his words, up to ten times. He was not treated by a specialist!

At the reception, the mother of an alcoholic: "And we have already turned to specialists with a license twice. But the treatment was unsuccessful." I ask: "And what recommendations did they give you?"

- Yes, there were recommendations. I was advised to do so-and-so.

- So you completed these appointments of specialists?

- No, I didn't.

- But why?

- Because I feel sorry for my son!

In this case, this is not about unsuccessful, but about the arbitrarily interrupted treatment and the refusal of the mother to cooperate with the doctor. Is the narcologist not sorry for her son? The main commandment of the doctor is, "do no harm." He would not advise that he could harm her son. Moreover, the recommendations from experts are always the same. Do not trust the doctor Paul, contact the doctors Peter, John, James, Andrew - and there you will hear the same recommendations. Do not trust doctors in your city; you will go to any other - and you will hear the same recommendations from specialists. Do not trust American doctors; you will go abroad for treatment - and there you will hear the same thing. Well, the doctors of the whole planet cannot be mistaken. Perseverance in upholding one's false views is one of the signs of co-dependence. I hope that I have tried enough to prove the validity of such recommendations.

Conclusion

So, you have closed the last page of the book "Quit Drinking: Easy Step By Step Guide to Stop Drinking Alcohol and Delete it from Your Life." You may have learned something new about yourself. Perhaps this book allowed you to look at yourself and the situation in your family from a distance. You saw yourself and your family as everyone around you sees, in whose families there is no alcoholism or drug addiction. Now you are faced with a choice. Before you are two ways.

One way - familiar and very convenient - let everything go on its own. To pretend that nothing happened, that everything that was mentioned above does not apply to you, and here is the basis:

- Firstly, you know your sick son (husband) better, better understand his condition than psychiatrists and narcologists. So, to carry out their recommendations, if you do not like them, is not necessary at all.

- Secondly, you are a perfect and infallible person. And if so, then you simply cannot make mistakes. Especially so large and serious, which can lead to your illness and even death of you or of a loved one.

- Finally, to change something in your life is so troublesome, so restless, and sometimes even painful. So it's better to leave it as it is - maybe it will resolve without your participation? And if it doesn't resolve and becomes completely unbearable, you will throw it in the trash, cross it out of your life and continue your sick ways? If, on the other hand, you read this book to find help for a loved one, maybe find yourself another person whom you will also love with your sick love, whose name is co-dependence?

True, there is another way - difficult, thorny, and new. The path that will ultimately lead your family to the big and bright road of a happy life, a life without drugs and alcohol. But then we must take responsibility for the fate and health of ourselves and our loved one on our shoulders. Then you must admit your own mistakes and, with the help of a psychiatrist-narcologist, do whatever is necessary in order to correct them.

If the justification of the proposed recommendations was sufficient for you and you yourself, realizing the degree of responsibility for the life and health of your loved ones, turned to a specialist for help and cooperate with him, strictly, consistently and accurately follow all his recommendations if, in case of difficulties and obstacles, you turn to the same psychiatrist-narcologist again, and do not change them one by one, succumbing to premature disappointment, then you are on the right track. With enough of your perseverance, with enough patience, the relationships in your family will become harmonious, and you, together with your loved ones, will be able to enjoy every day of life on earth.

And then look around. You will see that in some families of friends, relatives, and acquaintances, there are similar problems. Your happiness will not be complete if they suffer. Give them this book. Share your experience. Help them if you can.

In addition, your invaluable experience in curing alcoholism can be useful for many others in need, as you must have noted if you decided to follow the "Alcoholics Anonymous" method.

I wish you all the best in your endeavor!